Men's Sexual Health

This book is dedicated to my parents,
Mary Ann and James Samuel Peate.

Men's
Sexual Health

IAN PEATE BED(HONS), MA (LOND),
EN(G), RGN, DIPN (LOND), RNT, LLM
Principal Lecturer, Nursing and Adult Health,
University of Hertfordshire

W
WHURR PUBLISHERS
LONDON AND PHILADELPHIA

⌐ ∠ʋ03 Whurr Publishers Ltd
First published 2003
by Whurr Publishers Ltd
19b Compton Terrace
London N1 2UN England and
325 Chestnut Street, Philadelphia PA 19106 USA

British Library Cataloguing in Publication Data

A catalogue record for this book
is available from the British Library.

ISBN 1 86156 359 0

Printed and bound in the UK by Athenæum Press Limited, Gateshead, Tyne & Wear

Contents

Preface

In recent years, concern about men's health has come from various institutions and individuals – ranging from general political debates, social policy architects and the mass media, to the feminist, gay and men's movements. In this book, men are generally defined as males aged 16 years or older; younger males are also included where relevant. Some health problems are relevant only to men, e.g. prostate or testicular cancer; however, other health-related issues affect men more than they do women.

In a study undertaken by Dunn et al. (1998), a random sample of 1000 patients (both men and women) from four GP practices were asked about current sexual problems. The study revealed that men complained about the following:

- Difficulty getting an erection
- Difficulty maintaining an erection
- Either or both of:
  - premature ejaculation
  - sex never or rarely pleasant.

Approximately half the responders said that they would like to receive help for sexual problems; however, only about five per cent of those who wanted help had received it. Given an opportunity to choose from where such help would be most welcome, there was a preference for family doctor, family planning, well man clinic or trained marriage guidance counsellor. This study clearly demonstrates that men do want to receive sexual health advice; in fact, there is a high prevalence of sexual health problems and a gap between need and provision of service. Nurses, as highlighted in the study, are ideally placed to offer men help and advice.

For many men, the world in which they find themselves today is very different from the world in which their forefathers lived. Many aspects of their lives are different. Family life has changed. Nowadays more men marry later in life and marriage is still the most common form of partnership. However, separation and divorce have increased and many more couples are co-habiting before marriage. Nevertheless, and in spite of the changes in family make-up, families still play an important role in men's lives – family support and family contact are still common factors in many men's lives.

With regard to employment, specifically within sectors that have apprenticeship schemes, such as the motor industry and construction and electrical installation engineering, men outnumber women, whereas women predominate in such occupations as health and social care and hairdressing. There has been an increase in the numbers of men gaining qualifications in information technology areas, which may suggest that society is becoming more technological. A generation ago, it was unusual for men to study beyond the compulsory school-leaving age; now this is the norm. Although education results are improving for both younger men and women, the increase in females achieving better school levels and more qualifications is much faster than among their male counterparts. Women today are seen to accomplish more than men at various educational levels.

The established belief that the male is the family breadwinner is also being challenged with increasing numbers of women competing in the workforce, although women are still in the majority when it comes to part-time work.

Since the Second World War there have been many changes in the British economy. There has been a reduction in the number of jobs commonly associated with the manufacturing industries (historically this is where most men sought employment), with an equal increase in the number of jobs in the service sector. Many men are now employed in non-manual jobs, whereas a few generations ago they would have been engaged in manual work. There are still differences between the earnings of men and women – the weekly pay gap is wider than the hourly pay gap. This anomaly is because of the distinction between weekly and hourly pay; women tend to work on an hourly basis, whereas men are usually employed on a weekly or monthly basis. An additional reason may be that more men are employed in occupations where there is a greater possibility of overtime.

Men's health is almost a contradiction in terms. If men enjoyed good health they would not, on average, die when six years younger than their female contemporaries; even though there are more males born each year, men are consistently reported as living shorter lives than women. A male born in 1998 will have a life expectancy of slightly less than 75 years, compared with a female, who has a life expectancy of just under 80 years. When comparing females with males, men consult their doctors less often and are admitted to hospital more often than women. This last fact demonstrates that they have more serious health problems than women. Being a man can therefore have important implications – it can be a serious health hazard and should come with a government health warning! According to the International Covenant on Economics, Social and Cultural Rights (Article 122), all men and women have the right to the highest attainable standard of health. To fulfil this obligation, health policymakers must understand that men and women, as a result of their biological make-up and their gender role, have dissimilar needs, obstacles and opportunities (Meryn, 2002).

The most common cause of death among the male population is coronary heart disease; this is often linked to lifestyle. From a historical perspective men have tended to smoke more cigarettes than women; however, proportionally more men have given up smoking. The Government's recommendations on alcohol consumption are more often exceeded by men than by women. Men are 60 per cent more likely to be obese than women. Younger men eat less healthily; their diet has a higher fat content than that of older men or women. When considering physical activity, it is interesting to note that most men, and slightly more men than women, engage in at least moderate physical exercise, and considerably more men than women take part in vigorous physical exercise.

The single greatest cause of death in young males is suicide. When men attempt suicide it is more likely to be by using one of the more aggressive and violent methods. Men are also more successful in their attempts than women. *Our Healthier Nation*, a publication produced by the Government (Department of Health, 1999a), addresses four key areas of health – cancer, heart disease, accidents and mental health. This publication is particularly important for men because the four key areas impinge significantly on the health of the male population. Prostate cancer, testicular cancer, male breast cancer, coronary heart disease, accidents at work and as a result of high risk-taking activities, and suicide rates among men, especially among younger men, are all issues that nurses need to address when considering holistic nursing care.

Men commit most crimes, and are the major perpetrators of violence. Over a third of all male offenders are cautioned for, or found guilty of, handling stolen goods. Young men are most likely to become victims of violent crime, because they are more likely to find themselves in places or situations where violent crimes take place, e.g. pubs or football matches.

Inequality, whether characterized by social class, geographical area, ethnicity or gender, is a topic underpinning the work of the Health Development Agency (HDA). The HDA, a special health authority working to improve the health of people and communities in England and in particular to reduce health inequalities, has produced a report *Boys' and Young Men's Health* (Health Development Agency, 2001). The study provides an insight into the services available to boys and young men aged between 11 and 25 years. Gaps were highlighted between service need and service provision. Although there was evidence of much innovation in service provision (often nurse led), there still needs to be a more proactive approach to the services provided to men in general.

This book addresses issues of male sexual health from a variety of perspectives and contributes significantly to the overall provision of health-related services for all men regardless of age. The HDA's report stated that young men tend to access services when their condition (either physical or psychological) became much worse, especially when the fear of the issue with which they were confronted was bigger than the fear of appearing inadequate as a man. The key to addressing these issues lies in making access to services easier, e.g. providing young men with Internet or telephone advice and drop-in centres that are accessible, i.e. open when men can get there.

No matter what innovative practices are being used or developed and devised, the vital point is that these initiatives be subjected to rigorous research and evaluation in order to assess their effectiveness. There is clearly a lack of empirical research and evidence-based practice about men's health generally. The whole area has a dearth of research. Nurses are ideally placed to address this and to develop and construct databases to inform future practice. Although it is acknowledged that research into health, and especially sexual health, is often complex we must strive to put our nursing interventions to the test. We must discuss and make known examples of good 'effective' practice.

The report – *Boys' and Young Men's Health* – recommends that practitioners need to consider how they speak to young men who are seeking their help or advice. Nurses are in the forefront of helping to push the male health agenda forward and addressing the inequalities associated with male healthcare provision. The recommendations are that gender/masculinity issues be made more explicit. When nurses consider gender, they will be able to appreciate how some issues, e.g. suicide, are often gender driven. Furthermore, there are inequalities which may have been prevented if the gender issue had been addressed, e.g. the majority of people sleeping rough are men. Sex and masculinity are complex and will affect particular groups in a variety of ways.

Real interest in men's health is relatively new. During the late 1960s and the early 1970s, feminists began to develop radical views on society; this provoked a discussion and an awareness of their specific healthcare needs. They began to ensure that they had a voice concerning their health needs and started to challenge the patriarchal approach to all aspects of healthcare. It could be suggested that women have had their health needs addressed for over 20 years and that now men need to have their needs noted and acted upon. One aspect of this, an offshoot, could be that it allowed men to bring their needs for a health service to the forefront (however, this needs more debate). Men appear to feel that they have to be strong in mind and body, exemplify the image of fitness and be the household provider.

Men are often encouraged to be tough, hard and unfeeling, whereas women are often expected to be caring, tender and kind. This may continue to be perpetuated as long as society places pressures on men to conform to societal norms, i.e. what it is to be male.

Cultural stereotypes reinforce what is known as the 'male wound' (this debate needs more discussion than this text can provide). In this respect, it has been suggested that men go through two influential points in life at a very early stage – a splitting-up period. In the womb, testosterone is produced in the male embryo and this aids the conversion of a female pathway into a male one. Second, after having spent his life with his mother for the first three years or so, the male is then required to remove his identity from her and begin to identify with his father. This male wounding has the potential in later life to accentuate any problems that may arise in the family and other relationships that he forms. This biological sex difference starting *in utero* means that men are inherently at a disadvantage from the outset and will be more likely to fare less well psychologically than women. The male is again disadvantaged.

There have been several government health initiatives, e.g. the drive to modernize the NHS, the introduction of statutory bodies such as the National Institute for Clinical Excellence (NICE), and a commitment to clinical governance through the Commission for Health Improvements (CHI). The Prime Minister described the CHI in October 1999 as the boldest step yet to modernize the NHS. The overriding aim of the CHI is to ensure that every NHS patient receives the same high level of care. The Commission will eventually visit every NHS trust and health authority, including all primary care groups, local health groups and GP practices on a rolling process. Hence, men's sexual health needs will and should be addressed through the CHI and other governmental regulatory systems.

The National Service Frameworks (NSFs) also address issues that are pertinent to men. Four NSFs have been established so far; for older people, coronary heart disease, mental health and diabetes mellitus. Each NSF has implications for men's sexual health and each can be used to provide a framework for policy making and standard setting. All of these initiatives will strengthen the overall profile of men's sexual health needs.

There is no definition of what is meant by 'men's sexual health'; up to now, it has not been the subject of investigative research to any informative extent. There is no global definition of this concept. Yet, this is necessary because it would allow us to broach the subject in a broader manner than we do currently. We could maintain this breadth of definition to the advantage of our patients, e.g. by not pigeon-holing. We as nurses have to consider men from a social, political and economic perspective; to do otherwise would further disadvantage men. An advantage of this is to look at the whole being, not just from a sociological perspective.

Nurses are often mothers, fathers and partners to men as well as healthcare professionals, and as such we need to challenge our own perceptions of who men are and who we think they should be, and to take a new interest in men and masculinity. It will take many years for these feelings and images to be challenged and addressed, but we can begin to challenge them and prepare for the needs of current and future generations of males.

This book is for nurses in both institutional and community settings, who nurse people on a daily basis and who need to consider the complex sexual healthcare needs of men; it should be accessible for all nurses in the pre- and post-registration fields. Within the text you will find information that is readily available, accessible and easy to locate; it is hoped that this approach makes the book both user-friendly and readable. The text can be read as a whole or used for reference to clarify or reinforce specific issues.

Men must be actively involved in the decision-making process when it comes to the delivery of high-quality sexual healthcare. It is important that men's health issues be incorporated into health improvement plans. Local community plans should also consider men's health needs. Primary care trusts (PCTs) are in their infancy but it is hoped that each annual report prepared by the PCTs will comment on issues such as men's health. The contribution made by the voluntary sector as advocates should not be underestimated. Voluntary organizations are also in a position to monitor the activities of statutory bodies such as the NHS.

To develop a health service and policies that effectively meet the complex needs of the male population, nurses working in primary care settings, traditionally the GP surgery, must be prepared to devise alternative approaches. This could take the form of operating clinics in non-traditional settings, e.g. pubs, the workplace or barbers' shops. These approaches will mean that, at a grass-roots level, the needs of the people will be central to any improvements that are being considered by policymakers. The way forward, when considering men and their health needs, is in accord with Banks' (2002) lateral thinking.

Acknowledgements

I have been lucky to have had the support of so many people, and I should like especially to express my grateful appreciation to: my partner and best friend Jussi Lahtinen, my brother Anthony Peate, who contributed to many of the illustrations, and Frances Cohen.

.

CHAPTER ONE
Men's bodies

This chapter considers some central issues relating to the male body, e.g. gender and the concept of masculinity. It aims to encourage nurses to see the male not only as a physical entity but also as a psycho-sociocultural being. It sets the agenda for the rest of the text, demonstrating that men are complex beings with specific needs.

Nurses are asked to face the challenge with which they may be confronted when providing care for men. Care nurses are asked to provide for a wide and varied client group, and must be aware of the various factors impinging on men and their attempts to be healthy. To deliver high-quality sexual health care, nurses must confront any misconceptions, fears or anxiety that they have about their own sexuality or the sexuality of their client group.

Male identity is a very complex issue. Often, when nurses work with their patients, they become involved in a kind of bodywork of some sort; we communicate with our patients, even when we do not touch them physically. We do this using body language, gesture or with words. Social norms dictate distance in a social setting; however, when nurses are involved with patients in a therapeutic manner, they need to renegotiate these social norms, particularly when nurses are involved in sexual health issues; this is amplified even further when nurses work with male patients.

Hence, nurses are faced with new challenges when they attempt to help or to care for male patients with specific sexual health needs because, during this type of bodywork, the encounter has the potential to become sexualized (Heath and McCormack, 2002).

It is important to start at the outset by stating that there is a difference between what is understood by sex and gender. It is Kimmel (1995) who states that sex is the division between men and women, made on a biological basis. Gender is that which cultural meaning has ascribed to such biological differences. The biological attributes of being a man are therefore measurable and distinct from those of a woman. When nurses begin to apply gender issues to their patients, this is where the debate about nature versus nurture emerges. There are not only sexual differences in males and females; there are also issues such as culture and the concept of male identity. In this chapter, issues about sexual theory itself and the male are described. This is discussed in an attempt to highlight how, over time and subject to a changing social context, healthcare needs do differ between men and women.

The concept of sexuality is discussed and an attempt to define it presented. It is also important for nursing staff to understand the differences between sexuality and gender and also how difficult, if not impossible, it is to define these key terms.

A further discussion is presented about why, since the early 1990s, men's health has received more attention than it has done in the past. Nurses must address this very complicated issue from a holistic perspective in order to provide men with the high standard of care that they deserve.

Sexuality

Nurses must understand that sexuality and sexual health are an appropriate and legitimate aspect of nursing care; they have a professional obligation to address them. Some nurses may feel embarrassed about broaching the subject; when this is the case there may be many several reasons, including the following (RCN, 2000):

- Inadequate education about sexual health and sexuality at both pre-registration and post-registration levels.
- Personal views on sexuality, e.g. a hatred of homosexuality, or the use of contraception may be contrary to a nurse's own religious beliefs.
- Nursing culture may not regard sexuality and sexual health as important or appropriate, e.g. in elderly care settings.
- Lack of confidence, embarrassment and lack of knowledge may also prevent a nurse from instigating discussion about the topic.

There has been a plethora of literature over the past 20 years on the subject of sexuality. Wheeler (2001) considers the continuing discussion of sexuality within the realms of nursing and states that one document that has encouraged the debate has been *Sexuality and Sex Health in Nursing Practice*, produced by the Royal College of Nursing (2000). The Department of Health (2001) also encourages nurses to discuss and debate sexuality in its document *The National Strategy for Sexual Health and HIV*. Publication of such documents has the potential to raise the profile of sexuality and health care. Nurses are expected to treat the individual holistically, but until recently this could have been considered empty rhetoric, i.e. although the concept of holism was espoused it never really happened. The reason for making such a suggestion is that one aspect of the individual was often omitted – that of his sexuality. According to the RCN (2000), nurses are often wary of discussing sexuality with their patients because they received little education or training on the topic.

Sexuality is viewed in relation to such things as biology and the act of reproduction; this is not wrong but it should go further. Caplan (1987) and Brechin and Swain (1987) suggest that sexuality is a fundamental aspect of 'self'. Carr (1991) asserts that sexuality is the vehicle by which an individual will define him- or herself – it is central to his or her being.

The concepts of sexuality and sexual health have produced much debate over the years; they have also proved problematic for many health professionals in attempts to define the two concepts. One of the many reasons why these concepts bring problems is that society is constantly changing, which brings with it new definitions of social norms and societal boundaries. Sex and sexuality are complex spheres of human experience. Expectations of ourselves and others are in a constant state of flux.

One definition of sexual health often cited is by the World Health Organization (WHO, 1975):

> . . . the integration of somatic, emotional, intellectual and social aspects of sexual being, in ways that are positively enriching and that enhance personality, communication and love.

Van Ooijen (1995) considers sexuality from a female perspective as:

> . . . a woman's expression of herself as a sexual being; it is integral to her being. Whether or not she is sexually active is not an issue. It applies whatever her sexual orientation and whatever her sexual state of health.

It could be suggested that such a definition would also apply to men; however, as this text demonstrates, encouraging men to have an awareness of their sexuality is often more difficult than with women.

Fogel (1990) considers sexuality from a psychosocial perspective, thus:

> . . . the way we individually and uniquely express and project our identity and interrelate our physiological and psychological processes which are inherent in the way we sexually develop and sexually respond, both to ourselves and others.

Fogel's interpretation of sexuality appears to be all encompassing. She includes the important issue of a life span/developmental continuum. Furthermore, this definition explicitly acknowledges the uniqueness of the individual and his relationship with others.

Although these authors attempt to define the term, the definitions are abstract or vague. Wheeler (2001) makes the point that authors generally appear to think that nurses understand the nature of the term.

Defining key terms such as sexuality and sexual health may also be problematic because a definition of a particular term may lead an individual to typecast or stereotype people to 'fit' the definition that has been given. Nevertheless, to begin to understand these complex issues, a definition must be sought to aid comprehension. Whatever definition is chosen it must be broad enough to consider the individual as an ever-changing entity in an ever-changing society; it must also be flexible.

As a result of the various definitions of sexuality and the fact that sexuality covers a wide range of topics, Carr (1995) proposes that nurses may feel uncomfortable because of a lack of understanding when encouraged to broach the subject with men. Sexuality is an important topic and must be seen to be important to nurses because, as Sheerin and Sine (1999) suggest, it should be used as the main focus for holistic nursing care.

Sexuality is therefore a perplexing topic and is also very broad in its remit – covering diverse phenomena. It is concerned with biology and reproduction, but extends further to encompass the notion of 'self'.

Masculinity and gender

According to Hearn (1994), gender is a fluid concept influenced by social, historical and cultural elements, as opposed to anatomical factors. There is no biological reason why men should not wear dresses to work. Furthermore, there is no biological reason why men should not make good nurses or why women should not make good coalminers. Why these things are not common or the 'norm' is related to social and cultural expectations. These social and cultural assumptions about the sexes are what we call gender. Stoltenberg (1989) discusses social constructionist theories of masculinity and recognizes that gender is achieved through and by people, and the context in which they find themselves. Gender is not seen as something that we are, but rather something we engage in during social interactions.

From a biological perspective, sexual anatomy equates with sexual destiny. Male anatomy is confirmation of being a man (Moynihan, 1998). The world in which we live creates social boundaries and also causes divisions to be made. This is also true when we consider the roles that people play in society, i.e. whether they are masculine or feminine. The meaning of masculine and feminine are often context dependent and the messages they emit may be contradictory. Different groups ascribe different meanings to them – they do not mean the same things to members of different social classes, from divergent geographical areas and from distinct racial groups. Most societies assume that meanings associated with concepts such as masculinity are fixed, but this is not true because they differ across cultures and between people. Edwards (1997) does not rely on changing employment patterns to demonstrate how roles change; he considers the issue of male fashion and how, over time, through the medium of advertising, our preconceptions of what it is to be male are changing our attitudes. He suggests that male fashion and the manipulation of male sexuality in advertising campaigns have caused a rift between the traditional focus of male identity on work and production.

Men have various attributes, and the attributes they choose to express will be influenced by the context in which they find themselves. When in hospital, for example, they may feel that they have to control their emotions, but, when in a sports setting, e.g. on the football pitch, they may cry and hug their team mates (Moynihan, 1998).

The concepts of masculinity and femininity are not biologically fixed (Fulcher and Scott, 1999); they are socially constructed. Changing patterns of the social fabric shall and do dictate how such concepts are constructed and then deconstructed. It has often been said that the man is the breadwinner and provider for his wife and family. Changes in important social phenomena such as patterns of male and female employment are challenging such assumptions.

We divide the roles assigned to men and women in a variety of ways and over a period of time, e.g. from childhood to adolescence. Historically, men have been the centre of empirical and theoretical work (Maynard, 1999). Weeks (1993) suggests that, as a result of this, male dominance, 'maleness' and male sexuality have become the norm by which we judge women. I would suggest that this dominance also means that men are still classified by the concept of 'male' or 'masculine'; as such this brings many problems for men who do not 'fit' into the defined masculine role.

Males are expected to be strong and women are said to be more emotional. Being aggressive, being a rational being, having a need for control, engaging in competitive activities and being emotionally reticent equate to 'normal' attributes for a man (Edley and Wetherell, 1995). Moynihan (1998) states that ambiguity or contradiction is anathema to him. When men do not meet the sex role, stereotype problems arise. Being male and 'masculine' with a rigid, stoical stance adds to some of the physical and mental disorders that are disproportionately encountered by men (Kilmartin, 1994). The following are some of these masculine stereotypes:

- inexpressive
- aggressive
- ambitious
- analytical, assertive
- successful
- competitive

- forceful
- independent
- dominant
- strong personality
- athletic
- invulnerable.

In the early 1980s, Pleck highlighted that those men who do not conform to this societal 'norm' are in danger of trying to fit into the prescribed role with a negative effect on their mental health (Pleck, 1981). Making assumptions about men and their perceived masculinity may lead to care being delivered in an inappropriate manner. If we subscribe to one particular theory about men and their masculinity, this can have the potential to influence how we perceive phenomena and how we deal with them (Moynihan, 1998). Kilmartin (1994) points out that when we (healthcare professionals) equate masculinity with success, we only continue to perpetuate this Western myth. We are in danger of making it even more difficult for men to accept their illness, to seek help, and to express their fears and needs. Moynihan (1998) states that when men take illness 'like men should' this means that they will inevitably be hiding behind a brave façade, no matter how lonely or painful that illness may be. Hearn (1994) reports that men who consider themselves to be 'highly masculine' under-report symptoms. Motives and feelings are veiled when men report on the emotions they 'ought' to have, according to oppressive stereotypical myths of masculinity.

From the early years, we are promoting this masculine/feminine dichotomy every day of a child's life. We dress boys in blue and girls in pink. We refer to and treat boys and girls differently. Maccoby (1998) suggests that newborn boys were referred to as being 'sturdy', 'tough' and 'handsome', and girls as 'cute', 'dainty' and 'charming'.

Much early gender learning is done in a subliminal manner (Jolliff and Horne (1999), covertly. Early studies by Maccoby and Jacklin (1974) and Smith and Lloyd (1978) have highlighted that boys received reinforcements for being aggressive and girls for when they demonstrate signs of dependency. Boys are encouraged to engage in more physical activities than girls.

Masculinity and femininity are constructed in such a way that they are seen as polar opposites, so that we can understand that what men are, women are not, and what women are, men are not. To be a real man is to be seen as very different from women. Masculinity must not only be done, it must be seen to be done (Wilton, 2000). Reinforcement of the concept of masculinity at an early age, e.g. by encouraging male children to develop an emotionally detached role, may lead to boys having emotional problems later in life with their own children, their partners or their friends.

When nurses start to understand masculinity, we shall be able to target our healthcare initiatives more appropriately; we may also be better equipped to help men seek advice. Connell (1995) suggests that, at any one time, there may be a number of competing masculinities operating. If we are aware of this, we can begin to identify barriers that may be preventing our primary aim – to help and support men in a more effective manner.

The male body as metaphor

Hawkes (1972) describes metaphors as a number of figures of speech in which a word or expression is apparently used in other than its literal sense. Metaphors are central to our way of thinking (Savage, 1995) – they are essential conceptual tools that give meaning to our lives. As a result of this, the kinds of metaphor that we choose to use help us structure not only what we think, but also what actions we take (how we think determines how we act). Often, unconsciously, we tend to think a great deal in metaphors, i.e. conceptualizing one thing in terms of something else. We tend to shape our attitudes and our lives by the metaphors that we use (Grey, 1993). With this in mind nurses need to watch their words when communicating with men.

A metaphor is an important concept because words and ideas result in action. Salmond (1982) considers the power that metaphorical thought can have on each individual. She looks at how metaphor is often used in intellectual discourse. Intellect, through the examples given here, is seen as a journey, e.g. 'this starting point', ' from this it follows', 'we shall go further with our analysis' and 'and now we come to the end of our discussion'. In the context of men's health, Lloyd and Forrest (2001) use a metaphor – 'It is within this complex and rapidly changing territory that we have to look at the health of men and young men'; note the use of the metaphor 'territory'.

The metaphor often used for the male body is a machine; Watson (2000) refers to it as an 'organic machine'. An example of how this mechanistic metaphorical approach is used appeared in an advertisement produced by the Department of Health (1992). It was to promote its booklet *The Health of the Nation*. The advertisement pictured a well-oiled male in the position of Rodin's 'Thinker', and the internal organs of the man could be seen as the insides of a machine. The point of the advertisement was to encourage men to send for the booklet in an attempt to get them to make the first move to take some responsibility for their health. Watson (2000) suggests that the metaphorical image in the advertisement was that the male body is like a machine and that machines need looking after.

In this respect, health promoters are making many assumptions and reinforcing this virile image of the male. They may encourage men to engage in strenuous exercise regimens in an attempt to help them stay healthy; what they have not considered, however, is the link between the 'virile' male and morbidity.

Moynihan's (1987) study reveals how male clinicians often spoke to men with sexual health problems by using metaphors, e.g. infertility was referred to as 'shooting blanks' and unilateral orchidectomy, and the fear that there may be potential sexual problems, has been referred to as 'a plane flying with one engine and landing safely' or that 'one cylinder is as good as two'. Such type of talk can only reinforce the way men view their bodies as machines – controllable and controlled.

In Watson's (2000) work, he points out how men often use mechanical metaphors to describe body parts, e.g. the heart was referred to as 'a pump' and food as 'fuel'. Martin (1989) states that a mechanical metaphor is used by healthcare professionals to describe and dehumanize the physiological and psychological processes. The use of these metaphors imposes order on the body. Nurses must take care when using metaphors because they can often be a double-edged sword.

Men express their masculinity in many ways. When nurses are working with men they must take this into account.

Conclusion

This chapter has addressed some key conceptual issues about men, e.g. definitions of key terms and the concepts of gender and masculinity. It has highlighted the challenges that nurses may face when they aim to provide high-quality effective care.

Sexuality definitions are problematic. A consequence of this definition quagmire can be that nurses often steer away from discussion of sexuality with their patients. If sexuality continues to be defined in an impractical manner, nurses will continue to find it difficult to understand why sexuality is of particular importance to nursing practice. It is a topic that affects all of us and can be found across social classes. There is no one definition that addresses this complex concept. This, however, may be an advantage because we can begin to perceive sexuality and sex health in a broader framework, as opposed to a narrow, rigid, inflexible, single definition. There is little empirical evidence surrounding sexuality, and there is a need for nurses to undertake more research into all aspects of sexuality, for both nurses and patients

The concept of masculinity is also problematic; it has been stated that masculinity is a social construction rather than a biologically constructed entity. If we subscribe to the general theory that masculinity means one specific thing (i.e. to be masculine means that you have to be hard, to be brave and to lack emotion), then we are doing little to promote men's health generally. We should strive to think in broader terms. Stereotyping of masculinity will have many ramifications for the care we deliver to our male patients.

If nurses and their male patients continue to perpetuate the male gender myth, they are in danger of preventing men from talking openly and honestly about their health and illnesses. The image of a perfect man is often associated with the healthy man, which reinforces the issues of control and strength. A dilemma occurs for male patients as they become ill, because with illness comes a tainted perfect man; he may lose his sense of masculinity and with it his focus of control. The outcome can be detrimental to his health or recovery from illness. Nurses are ideally placed to counteract these dangerous stereotypical images.

CHAPTER TWO

Health education/promotion: a male perspective

This chapter considers various health education/promotion models and how practising nurses may use them to address the complex healthcare needs of the male population. The nurse is encouraged to address the health education/promotion issue from various perspectives, e.g. from an ethnic rather than an ethnocentric perspective.

Key issues are dealt with, e.g. what is meant by 'health' and how does a busy nurse devise health education materials that are to meet the needs of men? After all, it is important to consider sensitive issues such as ethics and politics when devising health promotion matter for men.

Many health promotion initiatives for men have been developed over the years. In this chapter nurses are encouraged to be creative and innovative in the health promotion programmes that they offer. Methods of evaluation of such programmes are outlined.

Definitions of men's health

It is demonstrated in this chapter, and others, that the term 'health' is, in general, difficult to define. There are many descriptions of what is meant by men's health but few definitions. Often authors consider mortality (Calman, 1993) or they will highlight particular conditions, risk factors and causes of death where, statistically, men are more likely to die, e.g. suicide rates, coronary heart disease, excessive alcohol use, drug use and accidents (Harrison and Dignan, 1999). In contrast, Sabo and Gordon (1995) begin with an understanding of men and then proceed on to the implications for health.

There is no agreed definition of what is meant by 'men's health' and, as Lloyd (1996) states, this may be one of the barriers to nurses discussing or taking up men's health as an important issue for the male population. Harrison and Dignan (1999) make a bold statement in their introduction, stating that it would be foolish to relegate the issue of men's health to disease

10

association alone; indeed they state that it would be a 'retrograde' step. What they fail to do is state what is meant by, or to define, men's health. This text offers several definitions and advocates that nurses use the definition that they feel is related to what the man in their care feels it should be. Therefore, men's health can be seen as a phenomenological issue.

O'Dowd and Jewell (1998) consider men's health to be associated with risk and a reluctance to seek help and advice, and what is meant by masculine behaviour. Fletcher (1997) provides us with a definition that is derived from a definition of women's health. In his adapted definition, he specifically states that men's health is concerned with conditions that are: unique to men; more prevalent among the male population; and more serious among men. It is also concerned with the different male risk factors associated with these conditions, and which different interventions are needed for men.

Lloyd and Forrest (2001) are content with a definition that is so broad that it allows for various conditions, behaviours, underpinning issues and differences in clinical practice, while still allowing a framework that is recognizable.

In summary, definitions are problematic but they allow us to begin to address pertinent issues about men.

Health promotion

Health promotion is relatively new. Naidoo and Wills (1994) suggest that, after publication of the Black Report in 1980 (Townsend et al., 1988), the importance of health promotion was brought into the limelight. The notion of health promotion first appeared after the WHO had announced its declaration of 'Health for All' in Alma Ata in 1978. The central component of primary health care in the Alma Ata accord was that community participation was essential – participation of the people will help to enhance the effectiveness of services. This approach also acknowledges the fact that communities will be empowered and involved in making decisions that will ultimately affect them. The traditional approach was to focus on methods to prevent disease and illness. The WHO (1986) defines health promotion as:

> The process of enabling people to increase control over and to improve their health.

Five essential components emerged from the first international conference on health promotion in 1986:

- Healthy public policy
- Creating supportive environments

- Strengthening community action
- Developing personal skills
- Reorienting health services.

According to Sutherland (2001), health is not merely the absence of illness or disease. Such a simplistic definition may be problematic: it may not encompass some values and beliefs that individuals hold close to them. Seedhouse (1986) suggests that a broader definition is needed and he states that a more positive approach should be adopted. Naidoo and Wills (2000) impart that there is no agreed definition of the term 'health'. Issues such as socioeconomic status, gender, ethnic origin and occupation will sway a person's concept of the term. Jones LJ (1994) confirms that health is a state of being that is subjected to wide individual, social and cultural constructions.

Health, suggests Naidoo and Wills (2000), has many associated dimensions, all of which need to be considered by the nurse (Aggleton and Homans, 1987). Figure 2.1 is a diagrammatic representation of the various dimensions of health.

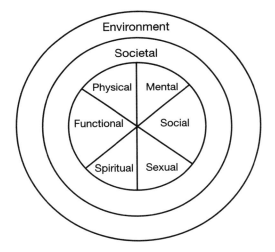

Figure 2.1 The dimensions of health (Naidoo and Wills, 2000).

Often the terms 'health promotion' and 'health education' are used interchangeably. Health promotion is seen as being broader than health education and having an element of social change associated with it (Denny and Jacob, 1990; Sutherland, 2001).

Methods of health promotion

Furber (1999) states that the term 'health promotion' may be described as an 'umbrella term' covering a variety of methods to promote health, with health education being just one of these methods. Other methods are those concerning public policy and have the potential to promote social change by improvements in living conditions, addressing employment problems, considering health and leisure facilities, and ensuring equal opportunities (Ewels and Simnett, 1999).

Health promotion models

As the concept of health is so elusive, it is not surprising that there are many different approaches to health promotion; this is evident in the different types and numbers of health promotion models available. One particular model is discussed here in detail.

It must be noted that models of health promotion are conceptual in nature and there are no hard and fast rules about how health promotion activities should be carried out. They are not guides to action, although they do attempt to describe the different underlying values and assumptions about health promotion.

There is no right or wrong approach to health promotion; much depends on the patient and the context of care and reflects on the different ways in which the nurse works. What does help, however, are models of health promotion or schools of thought. The model cited below is merely one of many. You could also consider the models of the following individuals: Tannahill (Downie et al., 1996), Tones and Tilford (1994) and Caplan and Holland (1990). These models help nurses to focus and make their own values and beliefs explicit based on a particular approach to health education. Naidoo and Wills (2000) suggest that they also help nurses to think theoretically about health promotion and can assist them in being creative and innovative in their health promotion activities.

The model that has been chosen has five approaches to health promotion (Table 2.1) and some more details are given below.

The medical approach

In this approach the overall aim is freedom from medically defined diseases such as testicular cancer, sexually transmitted infections or coronary heart disease. A paternalist approach may be evident here insofar as medical intervention is needed to prevent or improve ill-health. This paternalistic approach is often associated with persuasion, e.g. persuading men to use family planning clinics and consider screening for prostate cancer.

The behaviour change approach

The goal here is to alter individual attitudes and behaviours in an attempt to

Table 2.1 Five approaches to health promotion with sexually transmitted infection (STI) as an example

Approach	General aim	Health promotion activity	Important values	Specific aim and activity, using STI as example
Medical	Freedom from medically defined disability	Promotion of medical intervention to prevent or improve ill-health	Patient compliance with preventive medical procedures	**Aim:** freedom from STI and other health-related disorders **Activity:** encourage individuals to seek early detection and treatment of STIs
Behaviour change	Individual behaviour conducive to freedom from disease	Attitude and behaviour change to encourage adoption of 'healthier' lifestyle	Healthy lifestyle as defined by health promoter	**Aim:** behaviour changes from unsafe sexual activities to safe sexual activities
Educational	Individuals have knowledge and understanding, enabling well-informed decisions to be made and acted upon	Information about causes and effects of health – demoting factors Exploration of values and attitudes Development of skills required for healthy living	Individual right of free choice Health promoter's responsibility to identify educational content	**Aim:** patients will understand the effects an STI may have on their health; they will take the decision to perform safer sex activities **Activity:** giving patients information about the effects of unsafe sex activities; helping them to come to a decision that will reduce risk and to learn about safer sex activities
Patient-centred	Working with patients on his or her own terms	Working with choices of and actions for health issues, with which patients identify Empowering the patient	Patients are seen as equal Patients have a right to their own agenda Patient self-empowerment	Safer sex activities are considered only if the patient sees this as an area for concern The patient identifies what, if at all, he or she wishes to know about safer sex and what to do about it
Societal change	Physical and social environment which enables choice of healthier lifestyle	Political and social action to change the physical and social environment	A right and need to make the environment health enhancing	**Aim:** making unsafe sexual activities socially unacceptable, recognising the risks involved for all of society **Activity:** availability of condoms and lubricants in appropriate public places; promotion of safer sex for all members of the community

Adapted from Ewles and Simnett (1999).

encourage adoption of a 'healthy' lifestyle. (The definition of a 'healthy' lifestyle, according to Ewles and Simnett [1999], comes from the individual nurse or employer.) An example that is appropriate to behaviour change would be where the nurse encourages the patient to take up safer sex activities in order to avoid the risk of exposure to infection.

The educational approach
With this approach, the aim is to provide information, and assure knowledge and understanding of health-related issues in order to promote well-informed debate. The nurse presents health information about specific issues, e.g. the way in which to perform testicular self-examination, and the patient then decides whether he wishes to adopt new health practices. However, this approach means that the nurse providing the educational information must be knowledgeable, and he or she must also be flexible and able to adapt to the needs of the patient. Providing the patient with the appropriate knowledge means that he will be able to make an informed decision.

The client-centred approach
In this approach the nurse and the client (patient) work together on the patient's own terms. The patient identifies what information he requires and takes action (if he wishes) according to his interests and beliefs; the nurse facilitates this activity. The important principle underpinning this approach is patient empowerment; the patient is seen as pivotal to the process. Nurses and patients are seen as having equal status and each brings his own knowledge base, skills and attitudes (Peplau, 1952).

The societal change approach
In this final approach the objective is to bring about change in the physical, social and economic environment, with the end result being to make these more beneficial to health. The emphasis is not a change in the individual but a change in society. Health is an issue for all of us, from policymakers to individual nurses. If change is to occur and central Government policy is to change and consider the health issue more seriously, health issues must appear more within the political domain. We should encourage ongoing debate and dialogue so that individuals are able to make an informed decision when the time arises. According to Roper et al. (1996) major determinants of health are often firmly rooted in prevailing political, economic and social realities.

In this aspect of the chapter, we have considered one health promotion model in detail, which focused on five different approaches to health promotion: the medical or preventive approach; the behavioural or change of lifestyle approach; the educational approach; the client-centred, empowerment approach; and the societal change approach. Although we have dealt with each approach differently, in practice each one of them may and does impinge on the others. All the approaches discussed, however, have their own assumptions about health, community and change. Whatever model the nurse decides to use, she or he will need to be knowledgeable about the skills that she or he uses in order to put the model into action, and to have the necessary means of evaluating whether the chosen approach has had the desired effect. According to Naidoo and Wills (2000), by and large the type of approach adopted by the nurse will to some extent be dictated by the job, function and context of the care.

Health promotion activities involve various developments of a policy that has the potential to impinge on the health of those within a community. It therefore follows that politicians, civil servants and other government officials may become involved in health promotion, e.g. addressing or pushing for change in areas such as environmental health, instigating change through lobbying and becoming a member of community pressure groups. Ewels and Simnett (1999) and Naidoo and Wills (1994) feel that community pressure groups have become very much a part of the health-promoting process. In these cases community groups work closely with health promoters, although it is the health needs issues that they have identified which are developed and put into action, e.g. such groups as Gay Men Fighting AIDS (GMFA). GFMA has worked with health promoters to provide outreach work to men who have sex with men, encouraging safer sex techniques. The community group develops and grows, and in so doing generates feelings of control and empowerment.

This description of health promotion has demonstrated that a wide range of agencies can become involved in promoting the healthcare agenda. Health promotion therefore looks beyond the individual and considers the person's whole community and the environment in which he or she lives. Delaney (1996) describes this multi-sectoral approach as 'intersectional collaboration'. The main thrust of such an approach is to encourage communities to work together, in order to address issues that are of importance for all members of the local and national population. In *The Health of the Nation* (Department of Health, 1992), the Government demonstrated its commitment to communities working together by coining the term 'healthy alliances'. *The Health of the Nation* identifies collaborative alliances as working in various settings, e.g. schools, the workplace, hospitals and primary healthcare settings.

Health promotion and health promotion activities are complex issues that will encompass a variety of methods and activities, possibly involving many individuals, in order to achieve a change in public health policy. In the next section, the issue of health education is addressed.

Health education

The central aim of health education is to prevent disease by altering an individual's behaviour. *The Health of the Nation* (Department of Health, 1992) points out specific targets that are to be addressed in order to alter or change particular aspects of behaviour; individuals should be offered informed choices to help them adopt healthier lifestyles. This document was originally produced to address five specific areas of action: coronary heart disease and stroke, cancer, mental illness, accidents and sexual health. The successor to *The Health of the Nation* was *Saving Lives: Our Healthier Nation* (DoH, 1999b), and in this later document the area of sexual health was dropped because this was to become the focus of a separate strategy. The rationale underpinning the choice of the key areas was that they had to meet certain criteria (Mulhall, 2001):

- The area had to be a major cause of premature death or avoidable ill-health.
- Interventions that are proposed to address the key area had to be effective; there must be significant scope for improvement in health.
- Objectives and targets had to be set and progress made towards meeting these targets, and objectives had to be monitored.

The prevention of ill-health can be carried out in three ways, through primary, secondary or tertiary prevention (Table 2.2).

Table 2.2 Prevention of ill-health in respect of health education

Level	Aim	Example
Primary	Aimed at healthy people: to prevent ill-health and improve quality of health and life	Immunization, well man clinics, contraception, accident prevention, hygiene
Secondary	Aimed at those with a reversible illness, to restore health	Smoking, dietary changes, compliance with medication
Tertiary	Aimed at those with irreversible conditions, to limit complications and maximize potential	Rehabilitation after stroke; support for those with chronic conditions such as diabetes, asthma, emphysema

From Sutherland (2001).

Nurses are involved in all three stages of prevention and have an input at all levels. In primary health prevention, there is an attempt to encourage people to avoid illness; this can happen by detecting those people who are in the 'high-risk' group and providing these people with help and advice. For primary health prevention, nurses have a role to play in order to offer advice on the prevention of illness. Examples of this include well man clinics and the controversial issues surrounding immunization. Nurses are also well placed to offer both men and women advice about the most appropriate contraceptive methods available to them.

Secondary health prevention initiatives are challenging and also interesting. There are approaches here that we hope will, in effect, shorten the illness and prevent the progression of an illness, e.g. as nurses, we should consider how we offer advice about medication, how to promote issues about exercise, or even how to promote help for men with sexual difficulties such as erectile dysfunction.

Tertiary intervention attempts to limit complications or to limit any disability that may be the result of an irreversible condition or illness. In this aspect, nurses must look towards issues such as educating men about their disability and how they can form an opinion about their needs. Nurses can talk to those men with whom they have developed and established a nurse–patient therapeutic relationship about the opportunity to access many initiatives or the use of available rehabilitative services.

Male health promotion

Traditionally men are a very difficult group to provide health promotion for. There have been few health promotion initiatives for men (Furber, 1999), despite the inequalities associated with men's health. Fareed (1994) compared health promotion initiatives between men and women and concluded that those for women appear to stem from the 1960s and the emergence of the women's movement. Women, he suggests, questioned what services were available to them and, having done this, they made demands on health service providers to meet their specific needs. The result of this is the emergence of well woman clinics and screening activities. Women are able to access specific services allowing them to raise issues that concern their health, e.g. attendance at family planning clinics, prenatal and antenatal clinics; they are also much more likely than males to access immunization sessions for their children. Such activities are still hard to find for male health issues.

Marketing health

Health education materials are designed to promote lifestyle change, modify risk factors and meet the needs of specific population groups (Health Education Authority, 1997). Education about the effects of an illness, how to identify symptoms and when to seek professional advice from a nurse can play an immense part, in secondary prevention, in ameliorating the impact of a disease and preventing a recurrence (Coulter et al., 1998). Health promotion materials have been shown to have a useful effect on the uptake of screening programmes and the control of sexually transmitted infections (Healton and Messeri, 1993).

There are many ways in which information about self-care can be given; one recent innovation in the UK was the inception of NHS Direct (Department of Health, 1997). NHS Direct aims to give guidance to any of the public who have a health worry; health advice is available from registered nurses 24 hours a day, 365 days a year. Self-help manuals are available for those patients with chronic diseases such as asthma and diabetes mellitus. One such manual has been used as part of a programme to increase the sense of control and self-efficacy in people with arthritis, leading to an advantageous outcome (Lorig and Fries, 1995). Videos and multimedia packages can also be used, as well as the most popular method of information giving – the written word.

The Audit Commission (1993) undertook a study to determine the quality of communication experiences of patients and hospitals. Four groups of patients were used in the study – patients with benign prostatic hyperplasia, breast cancer, rheumatoid arthritis or stroke. This study uncovered a number of problems; patients:

- do not get written information about the condition, treatment or procedures
- get poor quality information
- get information too late.

There are, therefore, problems with patients being able to access information; the Audit Commission also made a number of recommendations in an attempt to ensure that accessibility of patient information would improve. However, to date there has not been a follow-up study that would determine whether these recommendations (Table 2.3) have been adhered to or complied with (Coulter et al., 1998).

As written information-giving is the most popular method of informing patients, it is important that nurses who prepare, design and distribute this information do so in the most effective manner. Greater accessibility of patient information is welcomed; however, it is of little value if the presentation and the content of the material are not of a high standard. What is important is that nurses ensure that they devise evaluative strategies that consider the readability and comprehensibility of the materials being used. The Division of Public Health and Primary Care (1998) has devised a tool that enables nurses to judge the quality of written material.

Table 2.3 The Audit Commission's recommendations for improving written information

Clinical staff and managers should work together to:
- Review current information that is currently distributed and the way in which it is distributed
- Determine what kind of information patients and relatives would like
- Provide written information about conditions, procedures and postoperative care
- Ensure that the written information available is deduced from national organizations
- Allocate both material and human resources for the production and purchase of written information
- Make sure that there are clear arrangements for the distribution of written information at the correct time, e.g. before a patient makes a decision about proposed surgery or before discharge from hospital
- Put in place arrangements for the proposals suggested above to be monitored to check efficacy

Adapted from the Audit Commission (1993).

Jadad and Gagliardi (1998) suggest that issues to be considered when designing health education materials include:

- accessibility
- acceptability
- readability and comprehensibility
- style and attractiveness of presentation
- accuracy and reliability of the content
- coverage and comprehensiveness
- references to sources and strength of evidence
- where to find further information
- credibility of authors, publishers and sponsors
- relevance and utility.

Developing effective high-quality patient information materials is not an easy task. It needs collaborative efforts from a wide range of people who have the expertise, including patients and their families, healthcare professionals, journalists, designers and editors. To provide good-quality information, Coulter et al. (1998) suggest consideration of the following:

- Involving patients throughout the process
- Including a wide range of clinical experts
- Being specific about the purpose of the information and also who the audience will be
- Considering minority groups and the information that they require
- Ensuring that the information presented is based on the best and most up-to-date material

- Planning how the materials are to be used
- Thinking about costs and feasibility of distribution
- Devising a strategy for distribution
- Evaluating the impact of the materials used.

To provide patients with information that will help them to make a decision, the nurse must consider these issues carefully. What is vital is that there is an evaluation/monitoring process in place to ensure that what is being distributed is also effective.

Well man clinics

On reviewing the literature, little has been revealed about well man clinics. Much of the emphasis in the early days appeared to centre on coronary heart disease screening, the discontinuation of smoking and excessive alcohol consumption. According to Webb (1999), there are many more issues that well man clinics can address. According to Robertson (1995), the 1980s saw the advent of well man clinics with a specific emphasis on screening men for illnesses such as cardiovascular disease and diabetes and giving advice to men to eat healthily and stop smoking. The differences between well man clinics in the 1980s and well woman clinics are that the men's clinics are often led and developed by healthcare professionals, whereas the well woman clinics have been primarily consumer led. The idea underpinning these clinics for men was to identify lifestyle risk factors, such as heavy smoking, that could later lead to ill-health. This was the opposite of general health clinics whereby the health professional identified a disease state and referral was made to a medical practitioner for treatment. As male morbidity and mortality are greater for men with heart disease and cerebrovascular accidents, cancers, mental illnesses and sexually transmitted infections including HIV/AIDS, and there are larger numbers of accidents, primary healthcare teams may consider setting up clinics specifically to target men. There are many ways in which well man clinics could be advantageous to men:

- Quality of care specifically aimed at men
- Healthier patients
- Male patient centred
- Meeting the needs of Government initiatives, i.e. a reduction in the number of cases of coronary heart disease
- Sensitive to men's needs
- Ideal opportunity for activities of sexual health promotion.

Webb (1999) asserts that health visitors who included clinics as a part of their weekly schedule originally set up the clinics. The venues for such initiatives varied and were often sited in local health centres or GP surgeries – the traditional places used by health visitors for clinics. In 1984, two male health visitors opened a well man clinic in Glasgow. In the following year, 1985, two male district nurses opened the first male family planning clinic in Manchester. The impetus for this initiative followed the publication of an important document *Men, Sex and Contraception* (Birth Control Trust and Family Planning Association, 1984). Funding for well man clinics came from a variety of sources, as is the case today. The funding arrangements for primary healthcare initiatives are complex and vary from county to county in the UK and from practice to practice.

Advertising the services of well man clinics

When advertising the services that well man clinics can offer, Webb (1999) states that the major way to do this is primarily through GP consultations, and advertisements in surgeries and health centres. Problems do arise with this form of advertising, however, so it is not surprising that the clinics are often poorly attended The main reason is that men do not generally go to GP consultations or (unlike their female counterparts) health centres. Those men who do not see the advertisements may be those who are in greatest need of the services offered by a well man clinic. Uptake may be poor because men perceive that the services are not for them. It may therefore be necessary to consider how and where the services should be advertised. Posters and advertising materials available in primary care environments often feature women and children; this approach lets users know that the service is specifically for them. Seeing these images, men may well feel that health-related services are not for them – but just for women and children; lack of appropriate male-focused issues may reinforce this notion.

Watson (2001) provides examples of how publicity for their well man clinic was carried out:

- Through women partners attending existing family planning and well woman clinics
- General practitioners
- Genitourinary medicine (GUM) clinics
- Local employers and job centres
- Libraries
- Pubs and clubs
- Local media.

A change is needed to ensure that men are explicitly included in advertising campaigns and that they are central to the campaign; an open and welcoming invitation should be also strived for. Some aspects of a well man clinic are (Watson, 2001):

- A free, personal and confidential service
- Timed appointments through a central booking service

- 'Walk-in' service
- Wide and varied range of services available
- Male staff available.

In one well man clinic, men cited several reasons for attending. A questionnaire was distributed asking new men why they were attending the clinic; 164 men completed the questionnaire of 168 men who attended the clinic. The study was carried out from October 1994 to September 1995 (Table 2.4).

Table 2.4 The reasons that men gave for attending a well man clinic

Reason for attending	Number	%
Free condoms	42	25.6
Information on HIV/AIDS	20	12.2
Information on STIs	16	9.8
General contraceptive advice	13	7.9
Information on vasectomy	12	7.3
Sexual or relationship problems	46	28.0
My physical development	25	15.2
Getting or keeping fit	43	26.2
Being fertile	9	5.5
Planning to be a parent	12	7.3
Health problems	51	31.1
Stress, depression and anxiety	48	29.3
Bereavement	6	3.7
Violence	6	3.7
Alcohol	10	6.1
Drugs	3	1.8
Giving up smoking	18	11.0
A health check – an MOT	99	60.4
How to look after myself	39	23.8
Anything else?	11	6.7
Total	**529[a]**	

[a]This total exceeds 164 because some men often selected more than one of the reasons that were listed.
From Watson (2001).

Practical issues need to be considered, e.g. where written information such as pamphlets/leaflets is placed; men may be reluctant to pick up leaflets in public areas such as GP surgeries or chemist shops. Nurses need to consider placing literature in private places, e.g. public toilets or sports room changing facilities. Placing the literature in such places may encourage men to read the information in private. However, Banks (2002) points out that placing leaflets in GP waiting rooms is an example of locking the stable door after the horse has bolted because many men tend to see their doctor late in the course of most conditions.

Appointment times

Men frequently complain that services are provided for them at times that are difficult for them (Davidson, 2001). Further issues also arise about consultations. As stated previously, some healthcare professionals tend to incorporate their sessions into the medical consultation or during the usual clinic routine. This may hinder the reason for the consultation and reduce its effectiveness, because the time allocated to an individual consultation may be short. Studies are needed to ascertain whether longer consultation times would indeed encourage healthcare workers to address and identify any necessary health promotion matters. Some men, however, may feel overwhelmed with a consultation that has been scheduled to last for up to 30 minutes, because they may be anxious about what may happen during the consultation. What the nurse needs to do in this case is give the man the choice of having a longer or shorter consultation as he sees fit; the nurse must ensure that the man is in control of the length of the consultation.

Staff gender

Is gender of staff important? Yes, it is important that the nurse gives due consideration to the gender of the staff who may run the well man clinic. Some men may state that they have no preference for either a male or female member of staff; however, some may state they would prefer a male, especially if the man has to answer sensitive questions or if he is to be examined physically. Furthermore, the man may feel that a female member of staff does not or cannot understand, for example, the language that he chooses to use to describe his problem(s), which may be intimate in nature. In contrast, some men can have the feeling that a female member of staff might be more sensitive to his needs than a male. The key issue is to be sensitive and attentive to the man's needs and to provide, if possible, a member of the same sex if he prefers. It should be noted, however, that this may present problems because there are more female staff employed by the NHS than male.

Brown and Lunt (1992) point out that, when nurses organize health promotion activities, e.g. going to pubs and places of work, they should be aware that it is often men in the higher social groups who access and make use of such services. Men from lower social classes are less likely to access them. In Chapter 3, the inequalities of health are discussed in more detail and implications of health and health service provision are highlighted.

Specific groups and health promotion issues

To categorize and 'pigeon-hole' men, e.g. ascribing them to a particular group – young, old, black, white, gay or straight – may be counterproductive. However, doing so may ensure that particular groups of male society receive care and support that is particularly sensitive to their needs. This aspect of the chapter does not intend to marginalize or isolate.

Lloyd and Forest (2001) consider that groups of young men fall into the following subgroups: black and minority ethnic men, gay young men, young men in care and young men who sleep rough. This list does not cover all subgroups, but it does highlight certain groups that may need specific attention. The subgroup's identity, e.g. young men who sleep rough, will have a bearing on the condition and theme that nurses need to take into account when planning services. The following gives a breakdown of what should be considered for each subgroup:

Black and minority ethnic men
- Mental health
- Sexual health and behaviour
- Suicide
- Help seeking

Gay young men
- Mental health
- Sexual health and behaviour
- Suicide
- Weight and eating disorders

Young men in care
- Mental health
- Sexual health and behaviour
- Suicide
- Physicality

Young men who sleep rough
- Mental health
- Sexual health and behaviour
- Suicide
- Risk taking
- Use of services.

When nurses are aware that certain groups of (identified) men are not managing well with specific aspects of their health, e.g. coping with mental health, they are in an ideal position to instigate creative and innovative health promotion activities.

The provision of sex and relationship education in schools is governed by policy. These policies help to guide school nurses and teachers to provide boys with useful and meaningful sex and relationship education. All schools have an obligation to define what is meant by sex and relationships and, furthermore, how these subjects are delivered. Teachers also have and will continue to have a vital role to play in providing schoolchildren with invaluable sex education. The Department for Education and Employment (2000) categorically state that the delivery of sex and relationship education is not the sole responsibility of schools. They say that others such as healthcare professionals should make a significant contribution. Many schools already work closely with healthcare professionals in the development and implementation of sex and relationship education programmes. School nurses have much to offer because they work closely with teachers and have much insight about referrals to local services such as family planning clinics, genito-urinary clinics and general practitioners. The school nurse can offer pupils a confidential service and provide support and advice, e.g. through organizing drop-in services. Although school nurses must work in partnership with teachers and parents, they have to follow their own professional code of conduct. Parents must be made aware of this professional responsibility.

Within the context of the prison service, nurses can also provide health promotion activities. There are over 67 000 prisoners in 137 prisons in England and Wales (Department of Health and HM Prison Service, 2001b). Many prisoners have sexual health needs and the prison nurse, like the school nurse, can provide advice and offer support to prisoners. It is noted that 8 per cent of all male prisoners are infected with hepatitis B and the figure is similar for hepatitis C. Approximately 0.3 per cent of the male prison population are infected with HIV. Of all prisoners 90 per cent have a diagnosable mental health problem (Department of Health and HM Prison Service, 2001a). The Prison Service is currently developing strategies that can help support prisoners to improve their physical and mental health, and bring the standard of prison health care to that offered in the NHS.

The Boys and Young Men's Sexual Health Team in Derby (Davidson and Lloyd, 2001) have targeted young men aged 14–19 years in areas where there are high rates of teenage pregnancy. Their work is undertaken in schools and youth clubs where high teenage pregnancy rates occur. They work with, and try to access, 'hard-to-reach young men' in places such as hostels and through referrals from the Youth Offending Team.

The aim of their work is to give young men the opportunity to discuss sexual issues by providing them with realistic and relevant sex and relationship education and to encourage young men to access male-focused health services. The methods used by the Derby Health Promotion Team to achieve the aims of the Derby project are:

- Male-only sexual health sessions
- Wide range of free and 'exciting' condoms
- Little or no waiting time
- A safe and confidential environment
- Participant-based sex and relationship education
- Encouraging young men to set the scene (programme)
- Use of sports activities to promote male health.

The underpinning assumptions when working with young men are to listen to their feelings and their attitudes and, having done this, regard their contribution positively. Nurses must try to remove or address the barriers that young men often feel prevent them from acting in a responsible manner, e.g. they may not want to have to travel to agencies such as family planning clinics for condoms, preferring perhaps to have them made available at youth clubs or hostels where they stay. It may be important for the group with whom nurses are working to discuss with or consult only male staff because this may encourage them to open up and talk.

The Derby project focused primarily on young white men. The From Boyhood to Manhood Foundation in London (Davidson and Lloyd, 2001) provided day, evening and weekend support services for African–Caribbean young men. Their target group comprised African–Caribbean boys and young men aged between 12 and 17 years in a large London borough. The main health issues addressed by the Foundation are:

- Educational needs
- Sexual health, including sexually transmitted infections and teenage pregnancies
- Relationships
- Diet and nutrition
- Physical health
- Social skills
- Behaviour modification
- Anger management.

The manner in which the Foundation addressed these issues focused on group work and individual work, and supporting parents; peer mentoring projects were also used. The target group was accessed via outreach schemes in the local community, and referral from other agencies such as schools and Youth Offending Teams.

When working with black men, an important underlying philosophy is to treat them with respect. Give them examples of other black men in society, their homes and their personal life who are functioning well. Skilled approaches must be developed that will nurture the will to alter hard and fast routines and to integrate young black men into the community in a favourable and positive way.

This work can be carried out by considering young black men in a holistic manner, from an Afro-centric viewpoint, so that the young men relate to and understand the aims of the project more meaningfully.

DeVille-Almond (2002) describes how her approach to men, encouraging them to seek help and advice, meant that she had to work 'outside the box'. She states that waiting for men to come to the surgery to seek help is not the answer; she advocates an innovative approach and takes her services to various male-dominated settings such as:

- A pub clinic
- Harley-Davidson 'pit stops' for men
- The Goodwood Festival of Speed
- GI's 'Big Boy' Clinic at the barber's shop.

In a small-scale study carried out by DeVille-Almond (2002), she explains that men do not access tradition GP services for several reasons:

- Surgery times make it too difficult to attend
- Receptionists are not approachable
- The surgery is more a place for women and children
- They would need to be really ill before bothering the doctor.

Results of holding the services away from the surgery revealed some very interesting findings from these men:

- Over 50 per cent had at least one long-term health problem
- Nearly half of those seen had obesity problems
- Associated with obesity, 62 per cent had hypertension
- Seven per cent were diagnosed with type 2 diabetes.

Holding a surgery is not a place for regular services. However, from time to time it is an environment that men coming to the clinic found convenient. In such venues, the opportunity arises to encourage men to think about their health and to highlight the importance of attending a GP surgery before they become seriously ill.

Johnson (2002) took her services to work sites and tied it in with a health day that was being run as part of the European Health and Safety Week. By taking the services to the site, the men could get themselves checked out more easily. Many of the men seen by Johnson (2002) used the opportunity to discuss personal issues that they were experiencing; for some, the issue that arose had never been discussed before. Many men stated that they were having individual problems with relationships; they often worked under short-term contracts and this type of work frequently took them away from home – the result was that they developed relationship problems and often had no GP to consult if they had a problem. The approach Johnson (2002) used demonstrated that imagination is vital if nurses are to create occupational health opportunities for men to access.

The practice examples cited above demonstrate two different approaches to how identified health issues can be addressed. It is important, however, to evaluate what the impact of such projects was on men's health, and whether the aims and methods used were successful.

There are other men in society, such as men with learning difficulties and men in prison or care, for whom nurses have a duty to provide health promotion. Hence, nurses must focus on ways in which to provide these men with meaningful sexual health promotion activities that reflect their specific unique needs.

Various evaluative methods are available to nurses – either internally by peers, e.g. internal audit, or externally by the funding body or one of the statutory bodies, such as the Campaign for Health Improvement (CHI). Dissemination of good practice should be encouraged because this may inform other nurses in the same field to provide effective care for men. Data such as the number of men who use or access a service, or the reduction in the number of suicides in a particular area, can be a means of quantitative evaluation. Qualitative evaluation, e.g. by interview, provides nurses with data that may be more subjective in nature, such as 'How do you feel about the services we offer here?' Pre- and post-programme questionnaires can help to evaluate the impact that a particular programme has had on participants' behaviour or understanding.

Conclusion

There are several definitions of health and there is no one correct definition; nor is any definition wrong. This also applies to health promotion models. Different people have different definitions depending on their own specific beliefs. These various definitions are likely to conflict with each other at some stage, depending on the situation in which an individual finds him- or herself, e.g. issues related to social class, gender, religion and occupation. These different interpretations of health come from a variety of perspectives, e.g. from medicine and the social sciences.

Nurses who are attempting to promote an individual's health must, first, be sure of the underpinning values and beliefs held by the patient. It is only when what is meant by health for that individual has been clarified that the nurse can begin to help the patient.

To involve men more in their health, the services currently offered need to be given further consideration. One main issue that needs to be addressed is the medicalization of the services currently offered to men; services should be provided that are client driven rather than service led. Taking services out to men appears to be one successful intervention.

CHAPTER THREE

Male health epidemiology

It would be unwise in a text about men's sexual health to ignore a discussion on men's health and men in general. It is vital that men's health is described from an epidemiological perspective, to acknowledge fully men and their needs in a healthcare setting. The data presented in this chapter are about men in general and the male health agenda from a variety of viewpoints. It is important to consider men from various perspectives such as age, marriage, divorce and living arrangements, educational achievements and employment because they may all have an overall impact on men's health. A comparative discussion about the various inequalities between men and women is presented.

A general discussion is presented about the documented inequalities in healthcare. Geographical variations – globally and nationally – are discussed. Data are derived from several reliable sources, e.g. the World Health Organization and the Office for National Statistics.

Many of the data given in this chapter about rates of occurrence are presented in relation to the incidence rates for women. In most of the incidences discussed, there is often a cause for concern because the incidence for men is higher than for women, e.g. drinking, deaths and not visiting general practitioners. This has the disadvantage, however, of comparison associated with competition and rivalry. This competitive edge – men versus women – is not intended to create a 'them and us' situation. However, by comparing men's and women's morbidity and mortality, this highlights or draws attention to the poor quality of healthcare available to men. Use of women's state of health as a benchmark must be done with caution, because it cannot be assumed that all is well with women's healthcare – this can create a false impression. It is, nevertheless, in the best interests of men and women that nurses strive to improve the quality of care for both genders.

Epidemiology

Epidemiology is the study of how diseases are arranged among various groups of people and the issues that affect the distribution of the diseases (Mulhall, 2001). Valenis (1992) suggests that epidemiology (the word is derived from the Greek: *epi* = upon, *demos* = people, *logos* = science) is the science of how and why diseases occur in various members of our society. The central concern of epidemiology is the who, what, where, when and how of disease occurrence.

Epidemiologists consider the experience of groups; they analyse differences between groups in order to establish whether there was a chance element involved in the different experiences, or whether these differences had an aetiological cause, and what was the aetiology or cause of the disease.

Most public health strategies rely on descriptive epidemiology, i.e. analysis of the distribution of disease, in order to plan and arrange for forthcoming health initiatives. The Social Focus on Men (Office for National Statistics, 2001) identifies and quantifies a wide range of data pertinent to men. The data presented in this publication cover a wider area than just health, e.g. lifestyle data – income, leisure and employment. The data presented illustrate different aspects of men.

As the term 'health' is somewhat obscure the data related to men's health are somewhat narrow. Mulhall (2001) suggests that epidemiologists use data-collecting techniques that will widen the current concept of health and incorporate lay perceptions and perspectives.

It is important to note that the data collected about men (from a variety of perspectives) should also incorporate a discussion on issues such as socio-economic factors, as well as the traditional biomedical causes of ill-health and male/female inequalities generally.

Inequalities in health

It was the Black Report 1980 (Townsend et al., 1988) that endorsed the fact that the different health experiences reported by people were indeed anchored in issues such as social class. The 'health divide' (Whitehead, 1988) suggested that socioeconomic factors appeared to be causing a major part of the health variations. This report also highlighted the fact that the health divide seen in adults across certain social groups had widened since the 1950s. Acheson (DoH, 1998) revisits such inequalities (e.g. social class and healthcare provision) in his report for the Labour Government. In this report he suggests that economic and social benefits of greater equality appear to go hand in hand. The quality of the social environment is at its worst when there is evidence of financial deprivation.

In *Our Healthier Nation* (DoH, 1999a), the current Government expresses its desire to deal not only with disease, but also with what causes those diseases. They cite issues such as poverty, inequalities, social exclusion, unemployment, and other features of the physical and social environment that converge to undermine health. In the search to identify why inequalities in health are apparent, policymakers will now have to consider social, economic and environmental issues, as well as the more traditional health-related behaviours such as diet, physical activity, sexual behaviour, smoking, and alcohol and drug use.

Other ways in which the Government wish to tackle the various health inequalities include involving local communities. They intend to place emphasis on a national contract for health, with the focus on working in partnership. The Government, and other national players, are seen as partners, with local players, communities and individuals all striving to work together to enhance the nation's health.

Policymakers are now alert to the fact that it is often difficult for an individual member of society to make a difference to the provision of high-quality healthcare and they are therefore concentrating on a partnership approach. Changes are more easily brought about if people work together – families, friends, and support from local agencies and the community as a whole. Without central Government leadership, local support agencies will be unable to carry out, and provide individuals with, support to prevent ill-health. Unless families, friends, individuals and communities work together the Government's aims and aspirations will not come to fruition (*Our Healthier Nation*, DoH, 1999a).

Epidemiology and heathcare professionals

For hundreds of years people have been trying to understand why certain diseases occur at particular times and why they are associated with some people at particular times. In the nineteenth century, Florence Nightingale tried to make sense of the infection rates she observed during her time at Scutari. Early public health initiatives also attempted to understand infection rates. Those investigators were originally sanitary inspectors. Arising from this was the role and function of the health visitor. During this period these inspectors and health visitors noted a link between environmental conditions and health outcomes.

In the late 1970s and early 1980s, the issue of the effects of socioeconomic factors on health began to emerge (McKeown, 1976), and a comparison was made between mortality and socioeconomic factors. At this stage, the issue of disease causation was related to multifactoral reasons. Health was now being seen more as a function comprising psychological, physical and social environments (Ashton and Seymour, 1991).

There have been many issues over the years that have promoted an increased awareness and acceptance of the findings from epidemiological investigation. Mulhall (2001) identifies three of these:

- Reorganization of the National Health Service, which was a result of the Griffiths Report (Department of Health and Social Security, 1983).
- Emergence of evidence-based practice.
- An acknowledgement that healthcare and healthcare provision are very closely related to a variety of socioeconomic factors.

The NHS has, since its inception in the 1950s, undergone much change and has had to adapt to many innovative and challenging ventures. Through an analysis of epidemiological data, a provision of quality care and a strategy to provide the appropriate services can take place.

The remaining part of this chapter considers men from a variety of perspectives. Epidemiological facts are presented on the following:

- Family life
- Educational attainment
- Employment
- Male health
- Lifestyle (including criminality).

Men and family life

It is advantageous to understand the size and structure of men in all aspects of society, including the labour market and various family relationships. This is because nowadays the types of family in which men live are increasingly disparate. Family structure is indeed changing, but the role men play is still important both to themselves and to their significant others.

Based on data from the 2001 Office for National Statistics, in the UK in 1999 there were 23.1 million men aged 16 or over; 17 per cent of these were aged 65 years or more (Table 3.1).

Northern Ireland accounts for the highest number of men who are aged between 16 and 24 years − 18 per cent. This compares with 14 per cent in the UK as a whole.

It should be noted that there was a high mortality rate in the male population over the age of 60 years in 1971, which can be attributed partly to the consequences of their time spent as soldiers in the First World War. It can also be stated that men aged over 60 years at that time (1971) may also have experienced a lower standard of living and could also have had a poor nutritional status when compared with contemporary older males.

Table 3.1 The numbers of men by age and their country of residence in thousands

Age (year)	England	Wales	Scotland	Northern Ireland	UK
16–24	2753	163	295	110	3321
25–34	3918	206	388	131	4643
35–44	3720	203	386	116	4425
45–54	3268	196	329	97	3890
55–64	2475	157	256	76	2964
65–74	1908	125	196	54	2283
75–84	1060	69	98	28	1255
> 85	263	16	22	6	307
All men aged ≥ 16	19,365	1135	1970	618	23,088

Source: Office for National Statistics (2001).

During the 1970s, fertility had decreased; the result of this was that there were fewer males under 25 years in 1999 than there were in 1971. The average age of the male population is increasing (National Office for Statistics, 2001). It can be said that this increase may be a result of lower mortality rates specifically associated with the older age group. In the late 1940s women began to outnumber men.

The British ethnic minority population has a younger age profile than the white population, which results from past immigration and fertility patterns. Table 3.2 provides information about male ethnic groups. Immigrant groups from south Asia, for example, have more men than women. Of those who are of Bangladeshi origin, 54 per cent are male, compared with 49 per cent in the population as a whole. The main cause for this gender ratio is earlier single male migration. In the coming years, these gender ratios will converge.

Households in the UK are more diverse today than they were in the past. Changes in family living, e.g. leaving home, forming initial partnerships, marriage or long-term union, having children and, for some, divorce, separation, lone parenthood and children leaving home can have an effect on a man's overall state of health. Households and families are considered in the next section.

One of the main changes in family life over the past 10 years has been the fall in the number of people living as married couples and an increase in the number of people who are co-habiting. Most men live in a married couple family, although the proportion has been falling, with just over two-thirds of men in the UK living in this type of household. Co-habitation is becoming more popular; in 1986 it was 3 per cent and by 1998–1999 this rose to 9 per cent. Young men tend to leave the parental home at an older age than young women (Table 3.3).

Table 3.2 Male ethnic groups: by age 1999–2000[a]

	< 16 years	16–34 years	35–64 years	≥ 65 years	All males (100%) (10⁶)
White (%)	20	26	40	14	26.1
Black (%)					
Black Caribbean	23	30	36	12	0.3
Black African	34	32	31	N/A	0.2
Other black groups	57	27	15	N/A	0.2
All black groups	35	30	29	6	0.6
Indian	24	29	40	8	0.5
Pakistani/Bangladeshi (%)					
Pakistani	37	34	25	4	0.4
Bangladeshi	38	35	22	5	0.1
All	37	35	24	4	0.5
Other groups (%)					
Chinese	20	44	32	N/A	0.1
None of the above	33	33	31	3	0.3
All other groups[b]	31	35	31	3	0.4
All groups (%)[c]	21	27	39	13	28.1

Office for National Statistics (2000/2001). N/A: not available.
[a]Population living in private households. Combined quarters: winter 1999 to autumn 2000.
[b]Includes those of mixed origin. [c]Includes those who did not state their ethnic group.

Table 3.3 Adults living with their parents: by gender and age in percentages

Year	Men aged (years)				Women aged (years)			
	16–19	20–24	25–29	30–34	16–19	20–24	25–29	30–34
1977–78	93	52	19	9	87	31	9	5
1991	92	50	19	9	87	32	9	5
1995–96	91	54	24	11	85	36	11	5
1999–2000	86	53	22	10	82	37	11	3

Source: Office for National Statistics (2001).

There is also a trend towards men living alone, and there are many reasons for this, e.g. they may choose to do so, it may be a temporary arrangement or there is simply no other option available (Table 3.4).

Table 3.4 Number of men as percentage in one-person households by age

Year	15–29 years	30–44 years	45–64 years	≥ 65 years
1971	0.7	0.8	1.8	2.0
1981	1.1	1.4	2.1	2.7
1991	2.0	2.7	2.7	3.1
1999	2.1	4.2	3.5	3.3
2011[a]	2.2	4.8	5.3	3.6
2021[a]	2.2	4.8	6.5	4.6

Source: Office for National Statistics (2001).
[a]Based on 1996 household projections.

The number of men getting married in the UK has for the first time fallen over the past 30 years. The number has almost halved from 401 000 in 1970 to 205 000 in 1999. There has been tendency for marriage to take place later in life and this is reflected in the increased numbers of people cohabiting.

Over the past 20 years or so, there has been a trend for first marriages to last for shorter periods of time. Table 3.5 outlines the number of men separated within five years of their first marriage.

Table 3.5 Number of men separated within five years of first marriage: by year of first marriage and age at first marriage

| | | Age at first marriage (years) | | |
		< 25 (%)	25–29 (%)	All < 30 (%)
Year of marriage	1965–1969	6	9	7
	1970–1974	11	8	10
	1975–1979	15	12	14
	1980–1984	12	7	10
	1985–1989	18	8	3

Source: Office for National Statistics (2001).

Generally speaking, those men whose first marriage was at a young age were more likely to have separated from their wife within five years than those men who married at an older age. Despite the fact that the divorce rate in England and Wales is higher among men aged 25–29 years (31.5 per 1000 married men), men aged under 25 years have experienced the largest growth in divorce rates over the past 20 years or so.

With regard to parenting, mothers are often seen as central to the parenting process; however, attitudes towards, and expectations of, fathers are beginning to shift. Most fathers are married and living with their dependent biological children. There have been changes within family life, with some fathers not having married, or being no longer married or remarried. Attempting to identify data about fatherhood is difficult, because information such as the age of the father at childbirth is not easy to determine. These types of data are limited to those cases where there has been a joint registration of the birth. Table 3.6 demonstrates the mean age of the father at birth of the child, although it must be reiterated that these data may be flawed to some extent, because fathers' details are present only on a joint birth registration; a sole birth registration gives details only of the mother.

Table 3.6 The mean age of the father at child's birth (England and Wales)

Mean age (years) of father at birth in	1971	1980[a]	1991	1997	1998	1999
Births within marriage	27.1	27.8	29.6	31.0	31.2	31.3
Births outside marriage	28.0	26.1	25.9	27.5	27.7	27.8
All live births	27.2	27.7	28.7	29.9	30.0	31.1

Source: Office for National Statistics (2001).
[a]There are no data available for 1981.

Almost one in four babies is born to an unmarried couple who are cohabiting as a family. The marital status of lone fathers varies, with almost half divorced and about a quarter of them separated. Figure 3.1 describes the marital status of lone fathers (Spring 2000). There were a total of 161 000 lone father families compared with 1 463 000 lone mother families.

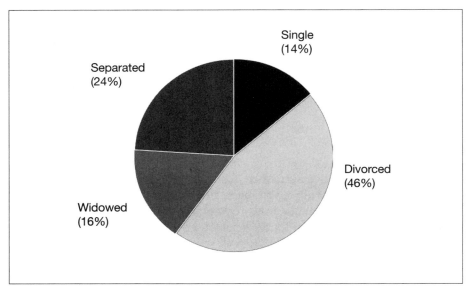

Figure 3.1 Marital status of lone fathers: Spring 2000.
(Source: Office for National Statistics 2001)

Men and learning

Within the population generally there has been an increase in the number of people continuing in education – many see gaining educational qualifications as a route to better social and economic success.

Younger men are more likely to hold professional qualifications than in the past. Those qualifications are often related to areas of information technology (IT) and the skills needed to compete in a society that is increasingly IT based. Nine of ten men in the UK in Autumn 2000, aged 16–24 years, held some form of educational qualification (Table 3.7).

Table 3.7 Highest qualifications held by men: by age – Autumn 2000.

	16–24 years	25–34 years	35–44 years	45–54 years	55–64 years	All men 16–64 years
Degree or equivalent (%)	8	21	19	18	13	17
Higher education (%)	4	8	8	9	7	8
GCE A level or equivalent (%)	31	27	30	32	33	30
GCSE grades A[a] to C or equivalent (%)	35	20	16	11	8	18
Other qualifications (%)	12	15	15	14	15	14
No qualifications (%)	10	9	12	16	24	14
All (100%) (10^6)	3.3	4.4	4.5	3.9	3.0	19.1

Source: Office for National Statistics (2000/2001).

When considering the highest educational qualifications held by men, other factors emerge, one of which is ethnicity. Fourteen per cent of white men of working age in the UK, in 1990–2000, held no qualification compared with 20 per cent from the Indian/Bangladeshi/Pakistani group. There is little difference in the numbers of ethnic minority groups and white men with degree qualifications.

Different types of job require various and different skills. It is often accepted that men who are in managerial, professional or technical occupations are more likely to have higher literacy levels than those men who work in occupations related to crafts and plant or machine operation, with plant or machine operators tending to have lower literacy levels (Office for National Statistics, 2001).

Low levels of literacy have a tremendous impact on an individual's life. The employment careers of men who left school at 16 and did not gain any qualifications were subsequently characterized by periods of unemployment. Furthermore, it has been suggested that fewer individuals with poor basic skills reported having good work-related skills, particularly in important areas of contemporary employment such as IT or computing (Organization of Economic Co-operation and Development, 2000).

Men are continuing to improve in their educational attainments, but women are improving at a faster rate than men, and are beginning to outperform men at various levels of education. It is interesting to note, however, that gender differences are apparent in subject choice, with more men than women still choosing such subjects as mathematics, engineering and technology.

Men and the labour market

Again, there has been a change over the past two decades in the roles that men and women play in the labour market. The proportion of men who are primary breadwinners has decreased, as reflected in the increasing numbers of women in the workforce. What does not appear to have changed is the differences in the participation of men and women in the workforce, e.g. there are still more men working full-time than women. In other particular occupations men predominate over women. There are many reasons for these changes in employment trends and types of work, e.g. changes in the global economy, new technology and international trading impacting on the jobs people choose, and ultimately male employment patterns. In 2000, 19.0 million males were of the working age, of whom 15.0 million were in employment. The UK has experienced much change since the Second World War: a decline in jobs in the manufacturing sector and an increase in industrial services.

Self-employment is also an important aspect of the labour force; it is estimated that in Spring 2000 (Office for National Statistics, 2001) over 2.3 million men aged 16 years and over in the UK were self-employed. This number increased from 2.0 million in 1984, to 2.7 million in 1990, and fell to 2.4 million in 1992. Self-employment is more common among men than among women; in Spring 2000 only 7 per cent of women were self-employed compared with 15 per cent of men.

In Table 3.8 the distribution of types of jobs between men and women is described. There has been a shift from manual to non-manual jobs; between 1991 and 2000, there was also a decrease by 4 per cent in the proportion of male employees who work in craft and related occupations, and a rise by 3 per cent of managers and administrators.

Unemployment has the ability to destroy a man's personal and social identity, specifically that of being the breadwinner and provider. This destruction of a man's identity and sense of self-esteem can have a catastrophic effect and lead to a life crisis, caused by, for example, increases in stress and anxiety. If a man loses his job, it has implications, e.g. for the provision of a balanced diet for him and his family. Lewis (1998) demonstrates that a man's mental health will deteriorate if he is unemployed and that there is an improvement in mental health if he returns to work.

Table 3.8 Employees by gender and occupation between 1991 and 2000

	Men (%) 1991	Men (%) 2000	Women (%) 1991	Women (%) 2000
Managers and administrators	16	19	8	11
Professional	10	12	8	10
Associate professional and technical	8	9	10	11
Clerical and secretarial	8	8	29	25
Craft and related	21	17	4	2
Personal and protective services	7	8	14	17
Selling	6	6	12	12
Plant and machine operatives	15	14	5	4
Other occupations	8	8	10	8
All employees[a] (100%) (10^6)	11.8	12.8	10.1	11.0

Source: Office for National Statistics (2000/2001).
[a]Includes all those who did not state their occupation.

Men and health

There are unacceptable inequalities in health in the UK, as established in the Acheson Report (Acheson, 1998). Death rates and life expectancy are key issues. Although death rates have continued to fall for both males and females (see Table 3.9 for death rates among men by age) across all social groups, there is a difference between those at the top of the social scale and those at the lower end. Inequality of life expectancy between social classes has increased over the past two decades.

Table 3.9 Death rates[a] among men by age (rates per 1000 men)

Year	16–24 years	25–34 years	35–44 years	45–54 years	55–64 years	65–74 years	≥ 75 years	All men ≥ 16 years[b]
1971	1.0	1.0	2.4	7.2	20.4	51.1	131.4	16.6
1976	1.0	1.0	2.2	7.2	20.0	50.9	135.8	16.7
1981	0.9	0.9	1.9	6.3	18.1	46.4	122.1	15.0
1986	0.8	0.9	1.7	5.5	17.0	43.5	117.2	14.2
1991	0.9	0.9	1.8	4.7	14.2	38.7	110.5	12.8
1996	0.8	1.0	1.7	4.2	12.4	35.4	106.8	12.0
1999	0.8	1.0	1.6	4.1	11.2	32.2	101.9	11.2

Office for National Statistics (2001).
[a]Data based on deaths registered each year.
[b]Age standardized to the European population.

Towards the end of the 1980s life expectancy for men in social classes I and II (the professional classes) was 75 years of age, compared with those in social classes IV and V (the unskilled manual classes) which was five years younger – 70 (Drever and Whitehead, 1997). Furthermore, when relating the social class of men to particular diseases, such as coronary heart disease, lung cancer, accidents, poisoning, violence, suicide and undetermined injury, there are particular differences.

Inequalities in health are evident throughout the population generally and among the various social groups; furthermore, this is apparent within and across gender and ethnic groups. The *Independent Inquiry into Inequalities in Health* (Acheson, 1998) stated that in the late 1970s, death rates were 53 per cent higher among men in lower social classes compared with those in the higher social classes.

Men are more likely to commit suicide, suffer from coronary heart disease, and have a major accident or drink much more alcohol than women. The expectation of life for males, as previously stated, is that they die earlier than women, e.g. those men born in 1998 will die aged about 75 years whereas women will have a life expectancy of 80 years. Such a gap equates to a similar life expectancy of males just after the Second World War.

The most common cause of death among men in the UK is circulatory disease, including heart disease and cerebrovascular accidents. In 1999 circulatory disease, accounted for two-fifths of deaths among men. After circulatory disease, the next killer is malignant neoplasms. More than a quarter of the men who died in 1999 had some form of cancer and, of all deaths among men, this was mostly from prostate cancer (Table 3.10).

Table 3.10 Main causes of death among men by age as a percentage, 1999

Cause of death	16–24 years	25–34 years	35–54 years	55–74 years	≥ 75 years	All men ≥ 16 years
Circulatory system	3	8	31	41	42	40
Malignant neoplasms	8	9	27	35	22	26
Respiratory system	3	3	5	12	22	16
External causes, of which:						
Accidents	35	24	7	1	1	2
Suicides and 'open verdicts'	25	27	8	1	–[a]	2
Digestive system	1	4	10	4	3	4
Mental disorder	10	10	3	1	2	2
Nervous system	5	4	3	1	2	2
Infectious diseases	2	2	2	1	1	1
Other causes	7	7	4	3	6	5
All deaths (100%)	2.5	4.5	22.8	107.1	160.0	296.9

[a]Negligible (less than half of the final digit shown). Source: Office for National Statistics (2001).

There are similarities between the numbers of men and women who die from circulatory or cancer-related deaths; what is interesting, however, is that when they are broken down into age groups there is a difference. The most likely cause of death for men is circulatory disease from the age of 35 years. However, when we consider women aged 35–74 years, the most likely cause of death is cancer. For both men and women diseases associated with the respiratory system are associated with a death rate of a fifth.

It is noted that there are age-specific gender differences in death rates at a young age. In 1999 there were twice as many deaths of men aged 16–34 years compared with women of the same age. Death rates that are particularly associated with accidents and suicides are far higher in young men than in young women. Of deaths in men aged between 16 and 24 years, 35 per cent were associated with accidents. However, when making a comparison in women, the death rate associated with accidents was 24 per cent, which may suggest that perhaps men engage in more risk-taking activities or behave in a riskier manner than women. Men are more involved in major accidents than women – see Table 3.11, which demonstrates the rates of major accidents in which men and women are involved.

Table 3.11 Annual major accident[a] rates (per 1000 men): by selected type of accident and gender, 1999

	Accident rates in men (%)	Accident rates in women (%)
At work[b]	10	3
Falls[c]	8	9
Sporting	4	2
Caused by a tool or other implement	4	1
Involving a moving vehicle	3	2
Any major accident	19	15

Source: Office for National Statistics (2001).
[a]Non-fatal accidents that caused the person to consult a doctor or go to a hospital.
[b]Per 100 men/women at work.
[c]Excludes falls while playing sports or exercising.

There was a conspicuous increase in the rise of suicides in younger men in 1999. In men aged between 15 and 24 years there were 16 suicides per 100 000 of the population; compare this with the suicide rate in the same age bracket in 1971, when there were only 7 suicides per 100 000 of the population.

It is interesting that there are differences in male suicide rates and marital status. The suicide rate in 1995 for widowed and divorced men aged between 15 and 44 years was 35 per 100 000 population, which is more than double the rate for men who are married. The incidence for single men has risen markedly since 1983 from 15 per 100 000 population to 22 per 100 000 population in 1995 (Office for National Statistics, 2001).

Generally speaking, despite their higher death rates and lower life expectancies compared with women, men are more likely to perceive themselves as having good health. Men often report having a sense of good health.

One in four men will die from a cancer-related disease, although one in three will actually develop cancer at some stage in their lives. Most cancers in men occur in the older age bracket. Less than 3 per cent of men aged under 40 years will have cancer; this increases to 81 per cent in men aged 65 years and over.

Since 1981, the incidence for the most common cancer in men – lung cancer – has fallen dramatically from 144 to 95 cases per 100 000 of the male population. This decrease is closely correlated with the number of men who have reduced or stopped smoking. The decline in the numbers of men who smoke is faster than it has been in women. Between 1974 and 1998–99, the proportion of men in the UK who smoked fell by almost half, from 51 to 28 per cent (Office for National Statistics, 2001).

After carcinoma of the lung, the second most common cancer in men is cancer of the prostate gland. In 1981, there were 48 cases of prostate cancer per 100 000 men in the UK. This number rose by 1997 to 82 cases per 100 000. Prostate cancer is a cancer that commonly occurs in older men; the incidence below the age of 45 years is very low (< 0.5 cases per 100 000 men). A sharp increase is, however, noted as age increases. In 1997 there were more than 700 cases of prostate cancer per 100 000 men aged 75 years or over (Table 3.12).

Table 3.12 Incidence rates for cancer of the lung, testis and prostate gland by age, 1997

| Age (years) | Incidence rate (per 100 000) of cancer of the | | |
	Prostate	Testis	Lung
15–24	0.1	5.8	0.1
25–34	0.1	13.4	0.4
35–44	0.3	12.1	5.2
45–54	9.6	5.1	35.8
55–64	92.2	3.1	145.9
65–74	337.9	1.4	398.8
≥ 75	726.6	2.0	626.0
All men aged ≥ 15	94.0	7.4	105.4

Source: Office for National Statistics (2001).

Although the incidence of prostate cancer is higher among older men, this is not the case with testicular cancer. Testicular cancer is more common among younger men, with those aged between 25 and 35 years being more likely to have the disease. Survival after cancer of the testis is now the highest survival rate for any cancer.

Coronary heart disease is much more common among males than females. It is associated with deprivation and there is a strong correlation between men aged 35–74 years living in a deprived area and the incidence of coronary heart disease (Office for National Statistics: General Practice Research Data, 1998). The more deprived an area in which the men live, the greater the chance of them having coronary heart disease. In men aged between 45 and 54 years, 21 per 1000 male patients from the least deprived areas were treated for coronary heart disease. This rate increased in those men living in the most deprived areas to 39 per 1000.

It is accepted that obesity, smoking, excessive alcohol consumption, hypercholesterolaemia, physical inactivity and hypertension are all associated with coronary heart disease. Therefore, men need to be encouraged to eat a balanced diet, reduce or stop smoking and/or drinking, and engage in physical activity.

Many of the data presented above have focused on physical health. *The NHS Plan* (Department of Health, 2000a) emphasizes the importance of mental health. The most common mental disorders were neurotic disorders such as anxiety, depression and phobias. In 2000, 135 men per 1000 were assessed as having some form of mental disorder; however, for women the rate is higher – 194 per 1000.

Sexually transmitted infections (STIs) have increased over the latter part of the 1990s. An explanation for this could be that there are more people undergoing tests for STIs or more people engaging in unsafe sex activities. As with coronary heart disease, there is a clear relationship between STIs and poverty. Diagnosis of certain STIs has increased, e.g. chlamydial infection, non-specific urethritis and human papillomavirus (the wart virus). Chlamydial infection rates have increased by 12 per cent (Stokes, 1997) in women and by 73 per cent in men. There are over 80 cases of chlamydial infection per 100 000 of the male population (Communicable Disease Surveillance Centre, 2001). There are also reports of outbreaks of syphilis (Communicable Disease Surveillance Centre, 2000). Knowledge about and awareness of some of the STIs are low. Half of the new cases of chlamydial infection in 1999 were among young men aged between 16 and 24 years, but when men of this same age group were asked about the disease 89 per cent of them had not even heard of it or did not know what it was.

The number of new cases of HIV that had been reported by the end of the 1990s had risen to a record level. Patterns of infection have changed since the early 1980s. In 1990, 13 per cent of new sexually acquired HIV cases among men were transmitted heterosexually; by 1999 this had risen to 31 per cent (Department of Health, 2001).

In 2001 central Government announced its strategy on sexual health and HIV services. This strategy is supported by an investment of £47.5 million to provide a range of initiatives set out in the strategy. The framework produced by the Department of Health for preventing the causes of premature death and ill-health has, as its key objective, to ensure that all individuals have access to the knowledge and skills necessary to acquire positive sexual health services, which should be readily available to all who need them (Kinghorn, 2001).

How often men use health and care services is a factor that has potentially large implications for the state of men's health. The use of NHS GP, inpatient and outpatient services rose across all age groups. There are, however, gender differences in those who access healthcare-related services. In the age group 16–34 years, the number of men who had consulted an NHS GP in the previous two weeks was half the number of women. There may be a reason for this, e.g. women often consult a GP for reasons of family planning and pregnancy. In addition, more women than men consulted a GP in the 35- to 54-year age group.

Interesting comparisons can be made according to the health service used by different types of men. Evidence suggests that men who are separated, widowed or divorced are less likely to report a good state of general health; only single men were more likely to report a good state of health than those who were married. GP consultations by men, their age and their marital status are provided in Table 3.13. Note that single men were less likely than other men to consult a GP.

Table 3.13 GP consultations[a] by men, their age and their marital status, 1998–1999 (percentages)

Age (years)	Single	Married/co-habiting	Separated/divorced/widowed
16–24	8	7	N/A
25–34	8	11	N/A
35–44	11	10	16
45–54	10	13	18
55–64	6	18	18
65–74	18	18	22
≥ 74	N/A	21	25
All men aged ≥ 16	9	14	20

Source: Office for National Statistics (2001).
[a]Percentage of men who had consulted a doctor (excluding a hospital) in the two weeks before interview.

Just as there are differences in GP consultations and men's age and marital status, there are also different consultation rates among ethnic minority groups: 22 per cent of Bangladeshi men, 17 per cent of Indian men and

16 per cent of African–Caribbean men had, in 1999, consulted a GP in the two weeks before being interviewed. Chinese and Irish men had similar consultation rates – 12 per cent (Office for National Statistics, 2001).

Male lifestyles

Leisure is seen as an important aspect of the lives of men. In 2000 about three in five men aged 15 years and over read a national paper. Data for the same year demonstrated that two in five men read a monthly magazine. In recent times new lifestyle magazines have emerged, which are often aimed at the younger age bracket and address issues such as health and fitness. Men engage in sporting activities more than women do. Participation in sporting activities can be a social activity as well as a way of getting and staying fit, and relieving stress. The more men are encouraged to undertake sporting activity, the more they can reduce illness.

Included in leisure is the issue of criminality. Although only a minority of men participate in criminal activity, men are more likely to be victims of most crimes than women. In 1999 male offenders made up over four-fifths of the total number of offenders in England and Wales. The number of male offenders, when expressed as a proportion of the total population, increases sharply in early adulthood and then, as age increases, decreases. The peak age of offending is 18 years, which accounted for 8 per cent of men who were found guilty or cautioned for an indictable offence.

The most common category of offence is theft and handling stolen goods. Drug-related offences are the second most common category. One in five male offenders is found guilty of this offence. Male offenders commit a wider range of offences than their female counterparts. Most women offenders are convicted of theft and handling stolen goods. Men, however, predominantly commit crimes of violence.

Men also are more likely to be the victims of crimes. Those at higher risk are aged between 16 and 24 years, which may be a case of being in places where violence commonly occurs, such as pubs and clubs. Other factors, apart from gender, may also have a bearing on who is a victim of crime, e.g. living in households located on council estates and with a low income. In these cases, the people are victims of burglary and violent crimes, which is not the case for those living in affluent areas.

Conclusion

This chapter has presented a great deal of epidemiological data. It is vital that nurses are aware of the epidemiological issues for men. To present a statistical picture of the experiences and lifestyles of men in the UK, the data must be set in context. This is achieved by making comparisons with women and considering men and their lifestyle experiences over time. The chapter has considered men from five particular, interrelated perspectives: family life, educational attainment, employment, male health and lifestyle, including criminality.

The world in which men live today is different from the world in which their forefathers lived, and many of the perspectives discussed here reflect these changes. The roles of men and women in society are changing and will continue to change. Family life is becoming more diverse; marriage is still the most common form of partnership but an increasing proportion of men remain unmarried. Women are increasingly making up a larger part of the workforce, so that married and co-habiting men are not necessarily the primary breadwinner within a household. Traditional roles in the home may still exist; men spend time playing with and caring for their children and, furthermore, they report that these aspects of family life are important to them. However, the sociological data suggest that in general, in most households, men still spend more time than women on traditionally male-oriented activities, e.g. gardening and DIY, whereas women are seen as the ones who do most of the domestic work.

Educational achievement for all young people is increasing and improving, although women's attainment has increased at a faster rate than men's. Both men and women are more likely to study beyond minimum school-leaving age. What remains steady are those men undertaking apprenticeships; they far outnumber women in the motor, construction and electrical installation industries. These jobs are often dangerous and may pose a danger to the health of men. Far fewer men work part time than women. Jobs that were traditionally based in the manufacturing industries are becoming fewer, and there has been an increase in the number of service industry jobs, accompanied by a shift from manual to non-manual work.

Men's health has recently received a great deal of attention. There have been many changes associated with healthcare, although men still appear to fare less well than women. Currently, men's life expectancy is five years less than that of women. The most common forms of death for men are coronary heart disease, stroke and cancer. Coronary heart disease is often linked to lifestyle; traditionally more men smoke than women, and men drink more alcohol. In addition, poor diet leads to more men being obese, and lack of exercise confounds the issue further.

Most perpetrators of crime are male, and the handling of stolen goods is the most prevalent offence, with drug-related crime second. Crimes of violence are almost exclusively attributed to men, and young men are more likely to be the victims of a violent crime.

Men's health is poor and the list below summarizes some of the most significant facts (Baker, 2001):

- The average male life expectancy at birth is currently under 75 years.
- The average man can expect to be seriously ill or chronically ill for 15 years of his life.
- Men who are defined as partly skilled or unskilled have a life expectancy of less than 70 years.
- Heart disease and stroke are, together, the biggest single cause of male deaths. The male death rate for these two diseases is 333 per 100 000 of the population.
- Indian, Bangladeshi and Irish men have higher rates of heart disease, and African–Caribbean and Bangladeshi and Indian men higher rates of stroke.
- Cancer is the second most common cause of male deaths, with a rate of 273 per 100 000 population.
- Nearly 22 000 men in the UK are newly diagnosed with prostate cancer each year and about 9500 die; the number of new cases diagnosed is expected to treble over the next 20 years.
- The incidence of testicular cancer has doubled in the past 20 years.
- The suicide rate among men is increasing.
- Depression is a widespread but under-recognised problem in men.
- Sexual problems are common among men: almost one-fifth of men in their 50s experience problems maintaining or achieving an erection
- Twenty-seven per cent of men drink more than the recommended limits; 36 per cent of men aged 16–24 drink excessively

Hence, society is changing and we are living in an increasingly diverse world compared with the lives our predecessors. Almost every aspect of a man's life has undergone a degree of change, much of which has been experienced by the most recent generation. Many examples of change have been depicted in this chapter: family lives are more diverse; health has, generally, improved; and changes are apparent in the labour market. Regardless of these changes, there are still health inequalities, and use of epidemiological data helps nurses to plan services that meet the needs of this population – males in particular.

Chapter Four
Testicular cancer

Compared with other malignancies, testicular cancer is a rare cancer; there are about 1400 cases each year in the UK. It is, however, also the most curable of cancers – 95 per cent of patients with testicular cancer can be treated. Testicular cancer tumours are very chemosensitive, which means that there is a high cure rate. However, Rosella (1994) states that 50 per cent of men with testicular cancer are diagnosed when the disease is in the advanced stages and prognosis is poor. Several men will therefore die needlessly from testicular cancer, because if treated early this disease can be cured. Many men do not perform testicular examination and there are many reasons for this. Nurses (in various clinical settings) are in an ideal position to teach and encourage men to carry out testicular self-examination (TSE). TSE takes only three minutes to perform; these three minutes may help to save a man's life. Survival is dependent on early detection, so men must be encouraged to undertake TSE on a 6-monthly basis. TSE gives men the chance to take responsibility for their own lives (Turner, 1995). The relative 5-year survival trends for testicular cancer in England, Wales and Scotland are outlined in Figure 4.1.

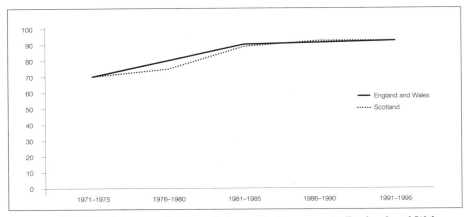

Figure 4.1 Relative 5-year survival trends for testicular cancer in England and Wales, and in Scotland. Source: Cancer Research Campaign (2001).

The group most commonly affected by testicular cancer – young men – is a perfect group for health educationalists and health educational strategies such as TSE. This group, despite the various health promotion initiatives available, is often misinformed about testicular cancer. Many men are unaware of or prefer to ignore it; furthermore, only 3 per cent regularly check their testicles (Orchid Cancer Appeal 1997).

Anatomy and physiology

The testicles are the chief male sex organs; they are not, however, the only male sex organs; they are equivalent to the ovaries in the female. The male reproductive tract also consists of the testes, their associated ducts, accessory glands such as the prostate gland, and the penis (Figure 4.2).

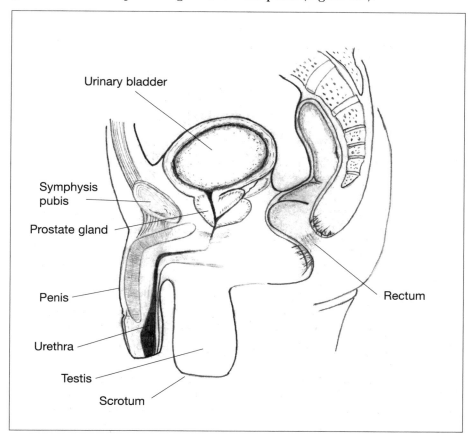

Figure 4.2 The male reproductive system.

The male has two testicles, which are oval shaped and about 5 cm in length and 2.5 cm in diameter. Each testicle weighs between 10 and 15 grams. Figure 4.3 shows the structure of the testicle.

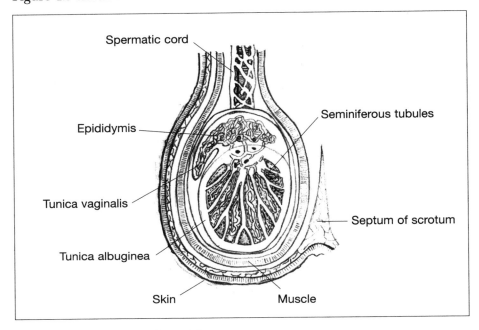

Figure 4.3 The structure of a testicle.

The testicles are responsible for the production of androgens and spermatozoa. There are two distinct cell groups that have responsibility for the production of androgens and spermatozoa: the Leydig interstitial cells and the Sertoli cells. The testicles are located outside the body in the scrotal sac. During embryonic life, the testes are developed from tissue near to the kidneys. Normally, a month or two before birth the testes usually descend through the inguinal canal in the abdomen wall and down either side of the scrotal sac. For testicular function to occur, each testicle must descend fully. The testicles are suspended from the external inguinal ring by the spermatic cord, which contains autonomic nerve fibres, blood vessels and lymphatics.

A constant temperature of 35°C must be maintained if sperm production is to occur, hence the external location of the testes in the scrotal sac. The testes are able to move up and down in the scrotal sac via a group of muscle fibres called the cremaster muscles, which allow the suspended testicle to shorten in order to maintain the required temperature of 35°C if the external temperature falls. The skin of the scrotal sac also has a role to play in maintaining temperature. The dartos muscle, situated within the superficial fascia of the scrotal skin, contracts when the external temperature falls, causing a dense wrinkling of the scrotal skin. When the external temperature increases, the muscle relaxes, and becomes flaccid and loose to aid cooling.

The blood supply to the testicles is from the testicular arteries. At the level of the renal arteries, the testicular arteries leave the aorta; they pass through the retropubic space into the groin, and then along the inguinal canal and down to the spermatic cord via the inguinal ring. Venous drainage also takes place along the spermatic cord; from there drainage passes to the left renal vein and on to the inferior vena cava. The pampiniform plexus, which surrounds the testes and epididymis, also facilitates drainage and it is thought that this acts as a heat exchanger to help maintain optimum testicular temperature.

Both testicles are encircled by two layers of tissue: the inner layer called the tunica albuginea (a fibrous layer) and the outer layer called the tunica vaginalis (a double layer). The outer tunica vaginalis evolved from the peritoneum and its function is twofold: to protect the testes from trauma and to sheathe the testes during intrauterine life. A small amount of lubricating fluid can be found between the two layers, which also helps to protect the testes from sudden movement. This cavity has the potential to swell and fluid accumulates in the space, with a resultant hydrocele formation. The tunica albuginea covers the testes and projects into the testicular tissue; this divides into about 200–300 wedged-shaped lobules. Within each lobule there are one to four convoluted tubules – the seminiferous tubules; these are the functional part of the organ. The seminiferous tubules come together to form a short, straight tubule – the tubulus rectus – which carries sperm into the rete testis. The rete testis is a network of tubules located on the posterior element of the testis. From here sperm are conveyed to the efferent ductules up to the epididymis.

Between the tubules there are groups of interstitial Leydig cells; these produce and secrete the androgens, e.g. testosterone; the androgens are secreted into interstitial fluid. After secretion, testosterone is absorbed directly into the bloodstream. The hormone testosterone has two primary functions. First, it maintains reproductive structures, including the development of spermatozoa; the second function involves the maturation of secondary sex characteristics that differentiate males and females. In the male, this includes a deeper voice, a greater percentage of muscle tissue and more body hair than in the female.

The epididymis

The epididymis is an elongated highly convoluted structure, packed tightly within each testicle; it is lined with secretory columnar epithelium. The epididymis is connected to the posterior surface of the testes. If uncoiled it would measure almost 6 metres. On palpation, towards the back of the testicle, it resembles a rough string-like mass. It is composed of a head, body and tail, which turns sharply upon itself and becomes the ductus deferens. The head receives sperm from the efferent ductules; storage is provided by the body and tail portions. The stored sperm are either ejaculated or, if ejaculation does not occur within 40–50 days, they begin to degenerate through a process of liquefaction and phagocytosis.

The vas deferens

The vas deferens is also referred to as the ductus deferens; it is approximately 45 cm in length. From the epididymis, it passes up into the pelvic cavity through the inguinal canal as an aspect of the spermatic cord. It then passes in front of the symphysis pubis, curves over the ureter and moves downwards, posteriorly, into the urinary bladder. The distal aspect of the vas deferens connects with the duct of the seminal vesicle that forms the ejaculatory duct. The duct passes through the prostate gland and then empties into the urethra. The vas deferens contracts rapidly during ejaculation and this forceful contraction ejects the sperm forward and through the urethra. There are three layers of muscle that help such forceful contraction; innervation of the muscle layers occurs through the autonomic nervous system.

Incidence of testicular cancer

Testicular cancer is the most common cancer and is the main cause of death in males aged between 15 and 34 years of age in the UK (Koshti-Richman, 1996). For all males, however, testicular cancer is rare and the most curable of malignancies. A correlation has been noted among the incidence of testicular cancer age, histology, geographical region and social class. Figure 4.4 demonstrates the incidence of testicular cancer per 100 000 population by age.

Men in the UK continue to be unaware of the importance and symptoms of the disease and the need to discover it early to improve the likelihood of survival (Katz et al., 1995). Furthermore, males who are most at risk (those aged 15–34 years) rarely practise TSE. Figure 4.5 outlines the number of new cases and directly age-standardized rates per 100 000 between 1979 and 2000.

The cause of testicular cancer is unknown (Cook, 2000). There are a number of risk factors that appear to be associated with the aetiology of testicular tumours; however there are few conclusive results, although there is an increase in evidence to suggest that environmental factors occurring early in life – probably prenatal – are important factors (Table 4.1).

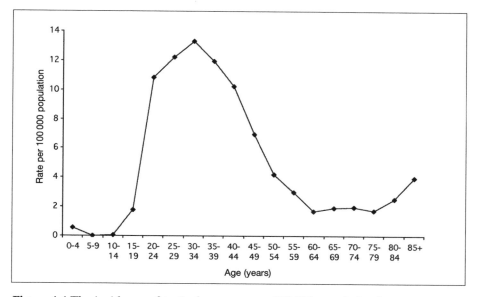

Figure 4.4 The incidence of testicular cancer per 100 000 population by age.

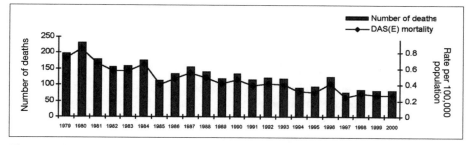

Figure 4.5 Number of deaths and directly age-standardized mortality from testicular cancer in the UK, 1979–2000. Source: Cancer Research Campaign (2001).

Men who have had cryptorchidism or testes that descend later in life are at risk of developing a testicular malignancy (about an 11–15 per cent risk); bilateral cryptorchidism carries a higher risk. Cryptorchidism is an established risk factor associated with testicular cancer (Cancer Research Campaign, 1998b). Although there is an increase in the incidence of cryptorchidism, this does not account for the increase in testicular cancer in the various populations around the world. The results of one study (UK Testicular Cancer Study Group, 1994) suggests that, for a man with a unilateral undescended testicle that has been successfully operated on (orchidopexy) before the age of 10 years, the risk of developing testicular cancer is reduced.

Table 4.1 Factors that may be associated with the aetiology of testicular cancer

Demographic factors	Age 15–34 years High social class White
Medical characteristics	First born Low birthweight Undescended testes Carcinoma *in situ* Previous testicular tumour Inguinal hernia Testicular torsion Mumps orchitis Early puberty
Prenatal factors	Oestrogen exposure
Genetic factors	Close family relative with testicular cancer Certain rare familial syndromes
Other	Lack of exercise Sedentary lifestyle Maternal smoking

Inherited genetic factors may play a role in a small percentage of patients. There are certain rare familial syndromes that are known to carry a higher risk; the same is true of a close family member who had or has testicular cancer. Dieckmann and Pichlmeier (1997) estimate that the relative risk for first-degree relatives of a patient is increased by a factor of 3:10. At least 2 per cent of all patients will fall within this category.

Carcinoma *in situ* is often found when the patient is undergoing investigations for infertility, on biopsy or after a diagnosis of testicular cancer. Over 50 per cent of patients with carcinoma *in situ* will go on to present with invasive carcinoma within five years and all cases over a period of 10 years (Jorgensen, 1990).

In certain medical conditions, risk is also increased. Infantile inguinal hernia increases risk two- to threefold; testicular torsion and a viral infection, e.g. mumps orchitis post-puberty, have all been positively associated with testicular cancer. A sedentary lifestyle and reduced physical activity may also increase risk (UK Testicular Cancer Study Group, 1994). Trauma, including sports trauma, is generally unrelated to the development of testicular cancer. This study also determined that there was no association for men who had undergone a vasectomy.

Exposure to high levels of maternal oestrogens during early foetal development could be the most common aetiological factor for many male reproductive tract disorders; these are increasing in number. Included in this are testicular cancer, cryptorchidism, urethral abnormalities and reduced semen, i.e. sperm count and volume (Sharpe and Skakkebaek, 1993).

Most cases of testicular cancer occur after the age of puberty; possibly the tumour is incited by the male sex hormones. Another important factor is that the average age of puberty is declining, which is in line with the increase in testicular cancer.

Geographical disparities

Although the rate of occurrence of testicular cancer is low globally, there appear to be discernible variations between certain countries. Ferlay et al. (2001) report that there were 49 302 incidences of testicular cancer worldwide and 8659 related deaths in the year 2000. Higher rates of testicular cancer are associated with men who are white and affluent; correspondingly, the disease has lower rates in men who are not white and from a lower socioeconomic class. The exception is New Zealand Maoris (see Table 4.2). It appears that men from northern Europe (although there are some discrepancies here) have a higher rate of testicular cancer. In non-white regions, the incidence is lower. In the variations noted between black and white men

Table 4.2 Geographical variations

Low incidence (< 0.2%)	Intermediate incidence (0.2–0.4%)	High incidence (> 0.4%)
Finland	Australia	Denmark
India	Belgium	Hawaii (white men)
Japan	Canada	Ireland
Poland	Czechoslovakia	Luxembourg
Portugal	East Germany	New Zealand (Maoris)
Romania	France	Norway
Singapore	Greece	Switzerland
South America	Hungary	
Spain	Iceland	
USA (black men)	Italy	
Yugoslavia	Netherlands	
	New Zealand	
	Sweden	
	UK	
	USA (white men)	

Source: Cancer Research Campaign (1991).

from the USA, in white males the disease is less prevalent; in non-white migrants there is no variation. It could therefore be suggested that environmental influences account for this discrepancy. The consistently lower rates reported with men who are black Americans compared with white Americans may also suggest a genetic component to the disease. The rates for Asian and Hispanic men are intermediate between those of white and black men.

Within Europe there is a distinct north–south divide. Rates in Denmark are five times higher than those in Spain and Portugal (Cancer Research Campaign, 1998b). It has been stated that higher rates of testicular cancer are associated with higher socioeconomic status. With this in mind, analysis of variations within England and Wales demonstrates that there are generally higher incidence rates in men aged 50 years or under in the south of the country, although this pattern is not entirely consistent (Swerdlow and dos Santos Silva, 1983). The pattern that has emerged would, however, be compatible with geographical variations. The geographical variation in men aged between 0 and 60 years is demonstrated in Table 4.2.

Histological variations

Germ-cell tumours (GCTs) account for 95 per cent of testicular tumours; of this, 4 per cent are lymphomas and 1 per cent is composed of disparate uncommon histological tumours. In men aged 40 years and over, it is usual to find lymphomas, which are often treated differently to GCTs.

GCTs are divided into two main groups: about 40 per cent are seminomas, with the remainder being non-seminomas, including malignant teratoma differentiated (MTD), malignant teratoma intermediate (MTI) and malignant

Table 4.3 Summary of the four main types of testicular malignancy

Teratoma	Accounting for 5–10% of all testicular cancers; more common in children and infants, but can also occur in the adult population
Seminoma	This is the most common type of testicular tumour; it has the best prognosis rate insofar as this type of testicular tumour is most responsive to treatment; this accounts for nearly a third of all cancers
Embryonic cancer	Accounts for a quarter of all cancers; it has a rapid growth and spreads quickly
Choriocarcinoma	1–3% of testicular cancers. Currently, this type of cancer has a poor prognosis associated with it

Source: Fillingham and Douglas (1997b).

teratoma undifferentiated (MTU) (Horwich, 1991). On average, teratomas occur 10 years earlier than seminomas, teratomas peak at 20–35 years and seminomas in the age range 30–45 years. Fillingham and Douglas (1997b) summarize the four main types of testicular malignancy in Table 4.3.

Symptoms

The most common symptom of testicular cancer is swelling in part of one testicle. This is often painless, although it may be associated with a dull ache in the lower abdomen or in the affected testicle. Some men complain of a feeling of heaviness in the scrotal sac. Other symptoms can include an increase in testicular firmness and an unusual difference between the testes. In some instances there may be a swelling and the testicle is very tender to touch (Cancer Research Campaign, 1998a). The disease is usually unilateral; bilateral disease is extremely rare (Raven, 1994) In advanced disease, some patients may present with the following symptoms: breast tenderness, shortness of breath, haemoptysis and low back pain (Cole, 1987).

Diagnosis and treatment

If a patient is suspected of having cancer of the testicle, he is referred to a specialist who will organize for a series of diagnostic tests to be undertaken. These include blood tests (to assess cancer markers), chest radiograph (to determine if there is any metastatic spread), computed tomography (CT: to assess lymphatic spread), magnetic resonance imaging (MRI) and ultrasonography.

Lymph-node spread occurs relatively early into para-aortic nodes and then on to the mediastinal nodes. Blood-borne spread commonly occurs to the lungs and liver (Neal and Hoskin, 1997). Figure 4.6 demonstrates the abdominal lymphatic system.

The treatment required to achieve a cure varies, depending on the type of tumour and the staging of the disease at diagnosis (Laker, 1994). It is therefore important that precise staging classification techniques are used, because this has an influence on therapeutic response. The variables affecting the outcome of treatment for testicular tumours are tumour size and serum marker levels. Delay in diagnosis correlates with the clinical stage of the disease (Hendry, 1999). Early diagnosis can also prevent the use of chemotherapy if the tumour is confined to the testes. Those patients who have metastases and high levels of serum markers will need an intensive regimen of chemotherapy (Horwich et al., 1989). Computed tomography is used to define the stage of the tumour and to detect whether there has been any

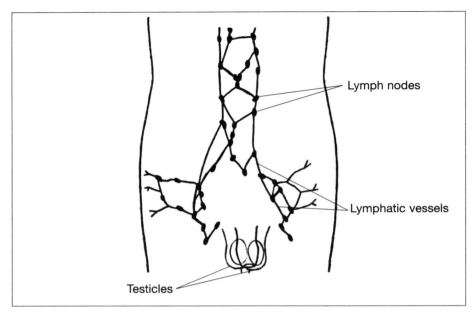

Figure 4.6 Abdominal lymphatic system. (Source: CancerBACUP, 1999.)

metastatic spread. A common method of staging testicular cancer is the Royal Marsden staging system (Table 4.4).

Besides staging of the tumour, blood is taken to assess the levels of α-feto-protein (AFP), β-human chorionic gonadotrophin (βhCG) and placental

Table 4.4 The Royal Marsden staging system for testicular cancer

Stage 1	Disease confined to the testes
Stage 2	Infradiaphragmatic nodal involvement (i.e. nodes below the diaphragm level) < 2 cm in size 2–5 cm in size > 7 cm in size
Stage 3	Supradiaphragmatic nodal involvement
Stage 4	Extralymphatic disease L1 Lung metastases > 3 in number L2 Lung metastases > 3 in number but < 2 cm in size L3 Lung metastases > 3 in number but > 2 cm in size H+ Liver metastases Br+ Brain metastases Bo+ Bone metastases

Source: Neal and Hoskin (1997).

alkaline phosphatase (PLAP). Three-quarters of non-seminomatous GCTs produce AFP or βhCG (Mason, 1996). The assessment of plasma levels of these particular tumour markers (produced specifically by cancer cells) not only allows for staging of the disease but also helps monitoring of treatment and detection of any subsequent tumour recurrence. Histological classification of the tumour is also needed. Table 4.5 demonstrates the histological classification of testicular tumours.

Table 4.5 The histological classification of testicular tumours

Seminoma	
Teratoma	TD: teratoma differentiated
	MTI: malignant teratoma intermediate
	MTU: malignant teratoma undifferentiated
	MTT: malignant teratoma trophoblastic
Combined tumour:	a malignant tumour, i.e. a combination of both seminoma and teratoma

After the Testicular Tumour Panel of Great Britain (Read et al., 1992).

There are three main treatment modalities: surgery, radiotherapy and chemotherapy; they may be used alone or combined.

Surgery

Orchidectomy may be the chosen line of treatment for men with testicular cancer. Surgery may have an important role to play in men who have been treated with chemotherapy for advanced non-seminomatous GCTs. Removal of the testicle allows for histopathological examination and the tumour can then be classified, which allows for further appropriate treatment to be planned.

Orchidectomy may be performed after testicular torsion or testicular trauma. The most common reason for performing unilateral orchidectomy is the presence of testicular tumours. Surgical exploration of the scrotal sac needs to be performed if the man is suspected of having a testicular tumour.

Hendry (1999) suggests that the ideal approach for examination of the scrotal sac is through an inguinal incision. In cases of a hydrocele obscuring the testicle, a scrotal incision would be indicated. If a tumour is evident, a second incision in the groin can be performed in order to remove the testicle and cord.

The procedure is performed under a general anaesthetic. Testicular biopsies for suspected tumours are not advocated when the contents of the scrotal sac are exposed, because there may be a possibility of tumour implantation in the scrotal wound and subsequent relapse.

Preoperative nursing care

The general principles of preoperative nursing care apply to patients who are to undergo orchidectomy (see Fillingham and Douglas, 1997b, for specific preoperative scrotal surgical care). What is needed, however, is a specific approach to the patient's psychological needs before surgery. The nurse needs to allow time for the patient (and his partner) to raise any issues. Advice must be given about fertility (see later for issues about the effects of treatment on a man's sexual health). Patients also need to be told by the nurse about the availability of a prosthesis, which, at a later date, can be inserted into the scrotal sac after the cancer has been removed. This can add to the aesthetics and a feeling of a fuller scrotal sac.

Postoperative nursing care

The patient should expect to be in hospital for at least five days after unilateral orchidectomy; this may, however, depend on the follow-up care needed.

There are two specific postoperative complications associated with bilateral orchidectomy: oedema and intrascrotal haemorrhage. Oedema around the scrotal area, resulting from the invasive nature of the surgery, can often be controlled by the application of ice bags for the first 12 hours and compression dressings for 3–5 days. Signs of haemorrhage may be directly or indirectly observed; the recording of vital signs and their appropriate interpretation can alert the nurses to a possible intrascrotal haemorrhage.

Bedrest may be advocated for the first 24–48 hours; however, early ambulation is advised according to the patient's condition. If bedrest is to be maintained, the nurse can help drainage of the abdominal/scrotal area by encouraging leg exercises. To try to reduce the degree of scrotal oedema, a rolled-up towel may be used to elevate the scrotum. To support the scrotum, an athletic support or tight underwear can be worn while in bed and when mobilizing.

When the patient is in the early stages of recuperation, i.e. when he is beginning to become fully mobile, the nurse can teach him activities that could prevent potential complications (Table 4.6).

Table 4.6 Teaching points for the patient who has undergone bilateral orchidectomy

---

Do not stand for long periods of time because this will increase scrotal oedema
Use an athletic support or tight underpants until healing is complete
Sit and soak in a warm bath three to four times a week
Avoid heavy lifting for at least 6–8 weeks

Adapted from Long and Glazer (1995).

Patients who undergo bilateral orchidectomy should be advised to refrain from sexual activity for approximately 4–5 weeks after surgery – including masturbation.

The nurse's role in helping the patient is to act as comforter, preventive agent, i.e. to help prevent complications, and educator (Roper et al., 1996). The environment in which the patient is nursed must be a supportive environment for both him and his partner. A knowledgeable nurse can correct any misconceptions the patient may have about the impending surgery and the outcome. Support is needed to help the patient come to terms with his altered body image; he may have feelings of being less attractive to his partner, because he is left with only one testicle, and may have feelings of inadequacy. Importantly, the nurse has to instil in the patient that he will need to attend the hospital for further follow-up.

Radiotherapy

Seminomas present with early stage disease and higher success rates are more likely with radiotherapy. It can be given to men who have already undergone orchidectomy to prevent recurrence of the tumour, or if there has been lymphatic involvement.

Radiotherapy for seminoma is a highly effective treatment; however, radiotherapy is not without its side effects. Common ones include nausea, malaise, diarrhoea and dysuria. It has also been noted that abdominal radiotherapy might be related to the formation of peptic ulceration (Neal and Hoskin, 1997). The side effects tend to last as long as the patient is undergoing treatment. It is important that the patient's nutritional status is maintained throughout treatment; it may be necessary to add nutritional supplements to the diet. Regular administration of prescribed antiemetics is an example of good practice. More severe examples of side effects associated with radiotherapy are bone marrow depletion; regular blood tests are needed to assess the degree of bone marrow damage; in some instances radiotherapy may need to be stopped and/or a blood transfusion given.

Chemotherapy

Chemotherapy plays a major role in the treatment of testicular cancer, especially if the tumour has spread beyond the testicle. For men with teratoma, chemotherapy is the most common choice of treatment, either to prevent a recurrence post-orchidectomy or to treat a diseased lymphatic system. Chemotherapy is deemed appropriate for men who have seminomas with metastatic lymphatic spread. There is one particular regimen that is often used in the treatment of testicular cancer – one that employs triple therapy of three chemotherapeutic drugs – bleomycin, etoposide and platinum (known collectively as BEP).

Chemotherapy can last for up to six weeks which could mean that the patient will need 3–4 days in hospital every three weeks or so. The duration of the treatment depends on individual assessment.

As some standard chemotherapy treatments may not be successful, or if the tumour is at an advanced stage, an alternative approach may be used. This involves the use of high doses of chemotherapeutic agents to destroy all cancer cells. There is a high possibility that the chemotherapy will destroy the bone marrow function as well. Peripheral blood stem cells may be taken from the patient before the start of the treatment. These peripheral blood stem cells can then be returned to the patient via transfusion after completion of chemotherapy.

As with radiotherapy, there are also potential side effects associated with chemotherapy. The major types of side effects are to do with the blood. The patient may have anaemia and be prone to developing infections caused by a leucopenia, resulting from blood cell death. If a patient develops pyrexia, this must be investigated and the cause determined; this may mean that the patient has an infection related to leucopenia. Antibiotic therapy may be prescribed as a prophylactic measure. Platelet depletion could also occur and nurses need to be observant, reporting any unexplained bleeding or bruising – a sign that the patient may have thrombocytopenia. Other side effects include nausea and vomiting, which may last for a few hours, and in severe cases several days. The use of antiemetics is advocated, as is the use of steroids. Careful monitoring of nutritional status is important.

Hair loss is one of the most common and most well-known side effects of chemotherapy, which can cause the patient much distress. Hair loss may be partial or complete. How much hair is lost depends on the type and dose of drugs used. If hair loss is likely to happen, it usually occurs within a few weeks of starting treatment; sometimes, however, this can occur within a few days of therapy. Patients also need to know that body and pubic hair could be lost. It is vital that patients are told that any hair lost as a result of chemotherapy will grow back once the course of treatment has been completed (CancerBACUP, 2001).

Effects of treatment on the man's sexual health

Unilateral orchidectomy does not affect a man's sexual performance or his fertility, if the remaining testicle is healthy. However, there are occasions when surgical removal of the abdominal lymph glands may be necessary – para-aortic lymphadenectomy – if they remain enlarged after chemo- or radiotherapy. This procedure can affect fertility because the sympathetic nerves are surgically divided and there is loss of ejaculatory function (Leiter and Brendler, 1967).

Most radiotherapy treatment has little direct effect on a man's sexual function. However, men who undergo radiotherapy may experience some sexual difficulties; there are many reasons for this. There may be loss of libido and impotence, which can be attributed to the fact that men are feeling very anxious at this time and have worries about the future, or that the treatment is making them too tired even to think about sex. Sperm production can be reduced in radiotherapy for testicular cancer and may lead to temporary or permanent infertility. Before undergoing radiotherapy, the patient should be given an opportunity to discuss his fears and anxieties. Sperm banking is an option that may be available for some men if the sperm are suitable. For successful cryopreservation of sperm, a particular number of sperm cells that are motile and capable of fertilizing an egg are needed; not all men have sperm that are suitable for storage. The practice and costs of sperm banking vary from hospital to hospital. Sperm can be frozen for several years until the couple are ready to have a family by artificial insemination.

Chemotherapy also carries with it possible sexual side effects. There may be a reduction in libido, and rarely there is pain on intercourse and difficulties with orgasm. However, fertility may be compromised. Infertility caused during, and for a time after, treatment is usually temporary. The rate at which the sperm continue to recover depends on each individual and usually returns to normal within 2–3 years. One in five men may have permanent infertility (CancerBACUP, 1999). The patient may also have poor self-esteem as a result of changes in body image, e.g. loss of hair (Stanway, 1995).

Testicular cancer can have an extreme effect on a man's concept of body image, especially as the testicles are closely related to the perception of being 'masculine', sexual vigour and the ability to father children. The combination of surgery, chemotherapy and radiotherapy can have an incredible effect not only on the man himself but also on his family. Nurses can provide men with the support that they need to help them cope with the many potential side effects associated with treatment for testicular cancer. The patient and his partner need a tremendous amount of psychological support and the nurse may need to refer the patient to a psychosexual therapist.

Health promotion

Given that there is a promising prognosis, as a result of early detection and subsequent treatment of testicular cancer, this emphasizes the importance of encouraging nurses to teach TSE. Rosella (1994) suggests that educational material be produced, but very little intervention material has been published on testicular cancer.

The nurse's contribution in terms of promoting TSE is another factor that can influence survival rates. By identifying those at-risk groups, as discussed earlier, the nurse is better placed to target and direct resources in an appropriate and meaningful manner. Paolozzi (1994) states that when the nurse promotes TSE he or she is improving men's health, reducing the number of deaths and illnesses, and empowering men. To do this effectively, nurses need to know which men are potentially at risk. According to Clements (1991) specific groups of nurses are in an ideal position to offer effective health promotion, namely practice nurses. Reeve (2002) suggests that school nurses, by using road shows to disseminate health promotion, are also ideally placed; such an approach raises awareness and encourages pupils to make informed choices on sexual health and relationship issues. The correct method for TSE is described in the Appendix.

The nurse is in an ideal position to continue to provide patients with a service that is unique to their needs. Currently, the subject of testicular cancer appears to be situated/located within the sphere of sexual health. Although there is no reason to discontinue such an approach, it must also be brought into a much wider domain. Nurses should engage in discussion with the patient when and where appropriate. It is not acceptable to ignore patients' needs because it is perceived that 'this is outside my area of practice'. If nurses continue to strive to provide holistic care, they must address clients' needs on a holistic basis.

Current health education and health promotion exercises may vary widely, with many resources being used to get the health promotion message across. Future challenges include improved public education, especially among young men, and greater awareness among the public in general and healthcare professionals in particular. As testicular cancer affects the younger age range, schools would appear to offer the ideal opportunity for health promotion. Carey et al. (1995) suggest that schools provide a 'captive audience'; in addition, it is recognized that health behaviours assumed during childhood appear to impact on adult health activity. There are, however, some concerns that need to be addressed here. Health education in schools is often left to teachers, who may not have any specialist training in this field; furthermore, there is no specific reference to testicular cancer in the National Curriculum. Effective education therefore depends on teachers' interpretation and interest. It would also appear that different schools give out conflicting messages, with some schools believing that school-aged boys are too young to be told about testicular cancer and TSE techniques (Peate, 1997). However, changes may be underfoot as described in the Government's recent publication *Sex and Relationship Education Guidance*

(Department for Education and Employment, 2000). This document calls for teachers to work with the wider community, i.e. school nurses in the provision of health education programmes that are school based.

Factors preventing effective TSE health education

Targeting young men and encouraging TSE at local and national levels are vital. However, there are many reasons why such an approach may be difficult, e.g. embarrassment (client/healthcare professional); lack of knowledge (client/healthcare professional), ineffective use of resources, and stigmatization. Lawler (1991) considers the subject of embarrassment in nursing interactions and associates this with the notion of taboo. O'Leary (2001) considers the issue further and suggests that some men may delay consulting a health professional because of the following reasons:

- Some men are afraid to confront the reality that their symptoms might involve.
- Men may not have enough knowledge about symptoms to relate them to their experience.
- Many men do not have the vocabulary in which to express their concern.

One major threat for men who may have testicular problems is in encouraging them to seek help. Young men are far more reluctant to consult a healthcare professional than are women. Men have little contact with primary healthcare services and this may have consequences for their future health. In the long term, this lack of contact prevents them from addressing their healthcare needs. Vital opportunities are missed when they do not seek help and advice, they do not have the chance to discuss health promotion initiatives and advice about preventive treatment is missed.

To defeat these problems, nurses must use an approach that the client feels is appropriate and with which he is comfortable. An anthropological approach could be suggested by gaining access to the client group and producing material that the group will understand and ultimately accept.

Recommendations for practice

Currently, there are some excellent approaches to encouraging young men to practise TSE. Although visual aids are helpful, there is room for improvement because most visual aids used tend to make use of line drawings to represent the man examining his testicles; a more 'realistic approach' – one with which men may more readily identify – could be the use of actual photographic images. It is suggested that this type of visual aid should be used to ensure that the message is clearly communicated, thus reducing ambiguity (Buggins, 1995).

It is imperative that the material used is context dependent, e.g. images that use white males for demonstrating TSE may be inappropriate for use in an Asian male youth club group, because this group would find it difficult to identify with the images. Helman (1996) highlights the problems that may be encountered when healthcare professionals' and patients' perceptions of needs differ. We are in danger of leaving our patients in a state of confusion and perplexity.

It is at this point that the anthropological perspective has much to recommend it. Teaching and learning sessions must be sensitive to the population under consideration. Language, as with images, must be adapted to the client group, to ensure maximum benefit. Buggins (1995) implies that, when nurses use language that patients do not understand, for example, this can leave patients feeling frightened, bewildered and undermined. Careful assessment of group characteristics will help to circumvent this outcome.

Responding to the needs of the client group is very important if the client is to be empowered and encouraged to contribute to his own healthcare needs. Williamson (1995) suggests that we must steer clear of a 'quick-fix' slant when attempting to modify behaviour; instead, he encourages an approach that not only responds efficiently to men's health issues but also exhibits social change. Luker and Caress (1989) suggest that the aim of health education/promotion is to produce a demonstrable behavioural change and change in attitudes. Specific groups of men must be identified, targeted, engaged, contained and empowered (Williamson, 1995).

Knowledge is the crucial issue. Nurses have this knowledge and must communicate it to their clients. Symptoms revealed early on in the disease warrant urgent attention. Men need to be able to recognize the early signs and symptoms of testicular cancer and to know where they can obtain appropriate advice.

When considering health education, nurses must listen to what it is that men want and they should be prepared to learn from the men for whom they care. There must be ongoing dialogue between men and healthcare professionals to take the issue of male health promotion forward.

Conclusion

The incidence of testicular cancer is increasing in this country. We are still unsure about the causes, and this may be a barrier to helping men prevent the disease. What is important is that we make men aware of the signs and symptoms of the disease, to encourage them to seek early help. Health professionals must be well informed, and react promptly by referring the patient to the most appropriate agency if early intervention is to become a reality.

By educating patients about their cancer, the required surgery and treatment modalities, the potential complications and side effects, and by providing continuous support and encouragement, we can help patients to address and work through their sense of self-loss and come to a more optimistic and positive outlook for their future.

Early detection and treatment mean that most testicular cancers, which 20 years ago would have killed young men, now carry an excellent prognosis.

Appendix

Testicular self-examination (TSE): your life in your hands

1. It is best to perform TSE after a warm shower or bath, when the scrotum is relaxed and the testicles are hanging lower from the body (it is normal for one testicle to hang lower than the other)
2. Standing in front of a mirror, visually inspect your scrotum for any signs of change – swelling or discoloration. Take your time and relax
3. Then place the pads of your index and middle finger of both your hands under one testicle and place the thumbs of both hands on top of the same testicle. Check one testicle at a time using both hands. Take your time and relax
4. Gently, squeeze your testicle and 'roll' it back and forth between your fingers and thumbs. Check the entire surface of the testicle while you do this
5. On the back of each testicle you will feel a small comma-like shape – the epididymis; this comma-like shape is normal. Check the epididymis for lumps. Towards the top of the epididymis you will feel the spermatic cord (vas deferens). Gently feel this for lumps and swellings too
6. When you have done this to the first testicle, move on to the other testicle giving it the same examination. Take your time and relax.

TSE should take place at monthly intervals; it only takes three minutes to perform a TSE. Following the steps illustrated will enable early discovery of any abnormalities. Diagnosis of testicular cancer usually begins with self-discovery. If you discover any abnormality you should seek urgent professional advice. Speak with your practice nurse/doctor; he or she can advise you.

What to look for:
• Pain, swelling and hardness of the testes
• Conversely, a painless lump on the testicle

- Heaviness in the scrotum
- Aching in the lower abdomen or groin area
- An accumulation of fluid in the scrotal sac
- A change in the way the testicle feels.

If you discover any of the above, speak with your practice nurse/doctor. Remember, these symptoms may not necessarily indicate cancer; there may be other causes for the above symptoms.

CHAPTER FIVE

Erectile dysfunction, definition and prevalence

Erectile dysfunction, traditionally termed impotence or erection problems, is a prevalent sexual health problem and affects a significant number of men and their partners (Keene and Davies, 1999). Downey (2000b) suggests that, in 21 per cent of cases, erectile dysfunction has been a contributing factor in the failure of relationships. Erectile dysfunction is seen as one of the most common sexual problems in men (Lobb-Rossini, 1999). As it is such a major healthcare issue, it deserves attention and appropriate treatment. It is problematic to come to agreement on a global definition of erectile dysfunction (Dean et al., 1999). Astbury-Ward (2000) reports that often it is the case that one definition of the condition is agreed on and, no sooner has this happened, than a change to that agreed definition is made. This reflects the rapid pace of change within the field. Lockyer and Gingell (1998) suggest that observations made by healthcare professionals are dependent on the definition used to describe erectile dysfunction. One definition that is most widely used is the definition provided by the US National Institutes of Health Consensus Conference (National Institutes of Health, 1993):

> Erectile dysfunction is the inability to obtain or maintain an erection sufficient for satisfactory sexual activity. It can be defined as the consequence of either organic or psychogenic disease. Erectile dysfunction is a complex interaction of them both.

It is difficult to assess prevalence because not all men will or are prepared to come forward and discuss such an intimate problem as an inability to attain and maintain an erection. Lobb-Rossini (1999) states that few men will live their lives without encountering an erectile dysfunction on at least one occasion. It is only when this occurs on more than an occasional basis, or causes distress to the man or his partner, that it becomes significant.

It is considered that in the UK there are over one in ten men who are affected by erectile dysfunction. This equates to some two to three million men in the UK.

Generally, erectile dysfunction is associated with, or more common in, men who are in the over-40s age group. As age progresses the complaint becomes more common. A study undertaken by Feldman et al. (1994) would suggest that men aged 40–70 years have a 50 per cent problem achieving and maintaining an erection. Men over the age of 80 years have a 30–50 per cent prevalence of erectile dysfunction (Carson, 1999). Despite the fact 10 per cent of men aged 40–70 years have complete erectile dysfunction, only a few of them will seek help and advice (Wagner and Saenz de Tejada, 1998).

Over 10 years ago it was suggested that erectile dysfunction was seen as a disease principally associated with or caused by psychological illness. Carson (1999) states that in the 1970s erectile dysfunction was often seen in men with a psychological basis for the condition. Recent studies have indicated that the physiology of erectile function and the pathophysiology of erectile dysfunction have altered this concept. Contemporary belief would suggest that those men who present with erectile dysfunction have an organic aetiology.

Erectile function of the penis is a complex function; it needs a combined neurological, endocrinological, psychological and physical (i.e. vascular) function. These functions are important for a positive erectile response. To understand the aetiological issues surrounding erectile dysfunction, the nurse should be aware of the mechanisms involved in penile erection.

The causes of erectile dysfunction may overlap and as such can be multi-factoral. It should therefore be reiterated that nurses must understand penile anatomy and the physiological response of penile erection.

Anatomy of the penis

The penis ('tail') is an organ of copulation designed to deliver sperm into the female reproductive tract. It is cylindrical in shape and contains the urethra for the passage of urine and semen. It consists of a body, root and glans penis. The body of the penis is made up of three cylindrical masses of tissue; each tissue mass is bound by fibrous tissue – the tunica albuginea.

The erectile apparatus of the penis is composed of paired vascular spongy organs – the corpora cavernosa; these are closely attached to each other except in the proximal third. Ventral to the penile shaft is the corpus spongiosum; the urethra passes through the corpus spongiosum, and then expands distally to form the glans penis. Penile skin is continuous with that of the lower abdominal wall; it then extends over the glans penis to form the prepuce and folds back on itself to reattach at the coronal sulcus. The shaft of the penis is enveloped in penile skin and, as the organ becomes erect, it can be moved freely. The dartos fascia is the underlying fascial layer and is continuous with Scarpa's fascia of the lower abdominal wall. Inferiorly, it continues as the dartos fascia of the scrotum and Colles' fascia of the perineum; it then attaches to the posterior border of the perineal membrane. The superficial dorsal vein lies within this layer of the fascia. The deep layer – Buck's fascia – covers both the corpora cavernosa and the corpus spongiosum in separate fascial compartments. Figure 5.1 details the fascial layers of the penile shaft.

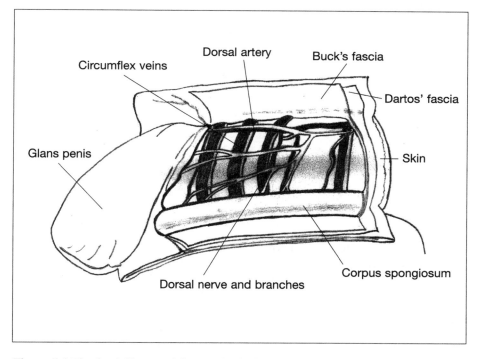

Figure 5.1 The fascial layers of the penile shaft.

The corpora cavernosa (the penile erectile bodies) are enclosed in a substantial fibrous sheath – the tunica albuginea (as stated earlier), which is relatively non-distensible and made up of elastic fibres and collagen that provide support for the rigidity achieved during erection. Within Buck's fascia (a gossamer layer of fascia), there is a complex vascular sinusoidal network of spongy tissue that stimulates erection. The two corpora are made up of mainly sinusoids containing smooth muscle tissue, which is lined with epithelial cells. The corpus spongiosum is also similarly constructed; however, this is enclosed by a less rigid, thinner tunica albuginea, resulting in less rigidity on activation (Figure 5.2).

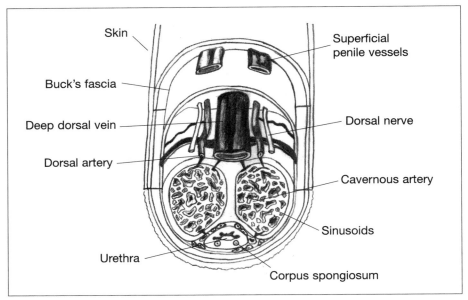

Figure 5.2 A cross-sectional view of the mid-penile shaft.

Blood supply

The blood supply to the corpora cavernosa begins from the internal iliac arteries and travels to the internal pudendal arteries; these terminate in the arteries to the penis. The penile arteries include the dorsal artery to the penis above the tunica albuginea, the bulbourethral artery travelling within the corpus spongiosum lateral to the urethra, and the central cavernosal arteries. They travel towards the central aspect of each of the paired corpora cavernosa and supply the blood for a successful erection.

Regulation of erection

For most of the time, the penis remains in a flaccid state; this is because sympathetic nervous impulses cause vasoconstriction of the arteries, resulting in a reduction of blood inflow. The first sign of sexual excitement is erection – the enlargement and stiffening of the penis. The penis may become erect in response to several sensations, e.g. smell, touch, sound, sight and thought. The primary responses, i.e. erection and detumescence, are through vascular events within the penis. Erection is not only a haemodynamic event, there is also a neurogenic element associated with it. The vascular events that occur are a fine balance between arterial inflow and venous outflow (Christ, 1995). The penis is in a flaccid state when arterial blood inflow is low and

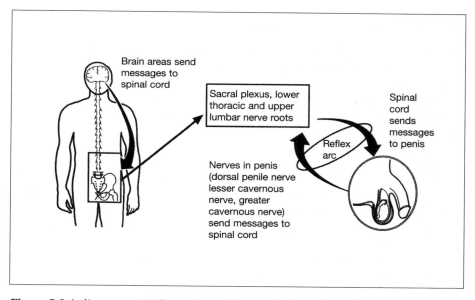

Figure 5.3 A diagrammatic illustration of the mechanism of penile erection. (Source: Nurse Education in Erectile Dysfunction (NEED). Pfizer Ltd., 2000.)

there is a balance with venous outflow; when tumescence occurs the arterial inflow will increase and venous outflow fall (Figure 5.3).

Dilatation of the cavernosal arteries is the primary event that leads to penile erection. The corpora cavernosa and the corpus spongiosum (erectile tissue) become engorged with approximately 20–50 ml of blood.

Central nervous system input can be stimulated or inhibited, and erection is under the control of the autonomic nervous system. Stimulation, especially in the glans or mechanoreceptors of the penis, activates parasympathetic nerves of the autonomic nervous system; several neurotransmitters are released, including nitric oxide, which causes relaxation of the smooth muscle in the walls of the penile arterioles. Nitric oxide is produced from intracelluar L-arginine. Endothelial cells release L-arginine and non-adrenergic, non-cholinergic neurons of the penis in response to sexual stimuli. In addition to the direct stimulation of the penis resulting in erection, there are some psychological factors that may have a significant effect on the erectile tissue of the penis, sometimes stimulating and sometimes inhibiting the erection.

There are three sets of nerves involved in normal male sexual function: thoracolumbar sympathetic, lumbosacral parasympathetic and lumbosacral somatic. Sensory fibres travel along the pudendal nerves to deliver penile sensation. Fibres transmit sensation centrally to assorted areas in the brain that control erection (Kirby, 1999).

Ejaculation and emission

Spinal reflexes send impulses to the genital organs and initiate emission when sexual stimulation becomes intense. The ductus deferens and the epididymis are thought to contract during emission, forcing sperm into the urethra. The seminal vesicles and the muscular coat surrounding the prostate gland contract and force fluids out from these glands. The glandular fluids and sperm mix with the mucus that is formed in the bulbourethral glands, forming the semen. It is this collection of fluids and the sperm in the urethra that represents emission.

When semen enters the urethra this causes nerve impulses to cross to the sacral region of the spinal cord; from here they cause rhythmic nerve impulses that supply the surrounding erectile tissue. Vasocongestion causes the head of the penis to increase in diameter and the testes to swell. Rhythmic sympathetic impulses cause peristaltic contractions of smooth muscle in the ducts of each testes, epididymis and ductus deferens, as well as the walls of the seminal vesicles and prostate gland. It is these rhythmic contractions that cause ejaculation of semen from the urethra. During this time the urethral sphincters contract, preventing flow of semen into the urinary bladder (Tortora and Grabowski, 1996). Accompanying ejaculation is the pleasurable sensation of orgasm. It should be noted that an orgasm and ejaculation are not one and the same thing; usually they occur together, but it is possible to have an orgasm without ejaculating.

Diagnosis of erectile dysfunction

The nurse may be the first person a man will turn to if he has erectile dysfunction and this may be in a hypertension or diabetic outpatient clinic. Although the patient may be happy to discuss his blood pressure or his diabetic management regimen, he may not feel too comfortable discussing or initiating discussion about his sexual problems. This may be the result of embarrassment or because he is unaware of the treatment options available. There are several known risk factors that will alert a nurse to suspect that a man is having erectile dysfunction problems. Once the nurse has been alerted to the potential problem, an assessment needs to be instigated; this allows the nurse to determine the cause of the problem and to plan future treatment with the patient and/or to refer.

Aetiology of erectile dysfunction

Originally it was thought that erectile dysfunction was psychogenic in nature; however, it is now recognized that certain organic causes are very common.

Each case of erectile dysfunction has an organic and a psychogenic component, but the balance between the two varies depending on each individual. Psychogenic erectile dysfunction can be addressed by psychosexual therapy and many patients have erectile function restored. In organic erectile function, it is unlikely for the patient to return to his normal sexual function unless there is some form of pharmacological or surgical intervention.

Psychogenic erectile dysfunction

Understanding the aetiology of erectile dysfunction means that the nurse must recap on the role played by the central and peripheral nervous systems in the physiological responses needed to achieve an erection.

The causes of psychogenic erectile dysfunction can be related to a variety of factors:

* Anxiety about sexual performance or sexual identity
* Anxiety that may be work related or associated with financial difficulties
* Psychosis
* Depression
* Sexual problems with partner
* Cultural, religious or social expectations.

Organic erectile dysfunction

There are many drugs (prescribed or recreational) that may induce or bring about erectile dysfunction. It must be noted, however, that there is very little empirical evidence to suggest that there may be a causal link between erectile dysfunction and the use of some drugs, although there appears to be a relationship between the start of drug therapy and the start of erectile dysfunction. If nurses are aware of these particular medications, they can be alerted to potential problems. The following are the drugs implicated:

* Antipsychotics/anxiolytics/hypnotics
  - Phenothiazines
  - Butyrophenones
  - Benzodiazpines
* Dopamine antagonists
  - Metoclopramide
* Hormones
  - Corticosteroids
  - Oestrogens
  - High-dose anabolic steroids

- Antiandrogens
  - Cyproterone acetate
- Anticholinergics
  - Atropine
  - Diphenhydramine
- Antihypertensives
  - Diuretics
  - Vasodilators
  - β Blockers
  - Angiotensin-converting enzyme (ACE) inhibitors
  - Calcium channel blockers
- Antidepressants
  - Tricylics
  - Monomine oxidase inhibitors
- Psychotropic drugs
  - Marijuana
  - Amphetamines
  - Alcohol
  - Nicotine
  - Opiates
  - Barbiturates
- H_2-receptor antagonists
  - Cimetidine.

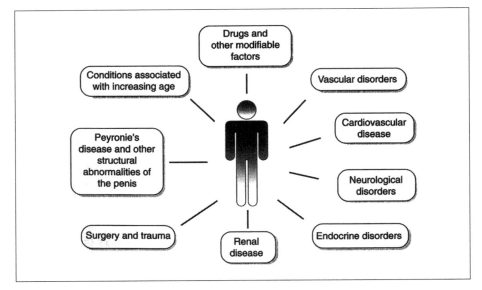

Figure 5.4 The aetiology of erectile dysfunction. (Source: Nurse Education in Erectile Dysfunction (NEED). Pfizer Ltd., 2000.)

Certain chronic illnesses that affect vascular and/or neurological supply to the penis are a common cause of erectile dysfunction, e.g. cardiovascular disease hypertension that coexists with smoking is associated with erectile dysfunction. Diabetes mellitus is also strongly linked to erectile dysfunction (Carson, 1999). Figure 5.4 summarizes the aetiology of erectile dysfunction.

Identification and assessment of patients at risk

As penile erectile function is complex, it involves a combination of satisfactorily functioning components of the human body. As a result of this the causes of erectile dysfunction often overlap and may be multifocal. There are many predisposing factors and conditions that have the potential to increase the possibility of coexisting erectile dysfunction. As such, the nurse must increase his or her awareness of these factors in order to identify those men at risk. These are the risk factors that need to be considered:

- Diabetes mellitus
- Cardiovascular disease
- Neurological conditions
- Surgery or trauma
- Anxiety disorders
- Depression or psychiatric disorders
- Drugs
- Tobacco
- Hormonal imbalance
- Relationship difficulties.

The impact of erectile dysfunction on a man and his partner can have far-reaching effects. The ability of a man to initiate and maintain an erection is considered central to his sense of well-being. The nurse must therefore bear in mind that problems associated with erectile dysfunction can have an effect on the man's (and his partner's) quality of life.

Many men will not have the confidence to approach a nurse about their erectile problems; the nurse may therefore need to initiate discussion with those individuals she or he suspects of being at risk. There are several circumstances where the nurse could discuss sexual activity:

- Genitourinary (GUM) clinic
- Well man clinic
- New patient healthcare check
- Hypertension/diabetic clinics
- Pre-employment occupational health assessments

- Female consultations such as family planning clinics, ante-/postnatal checks and cervical smear tests.

When a patient approaches the nurse in consultation about his erectile problem, the nurse must ensure that the patient understands what erectile dysfunction is. Emphasis must be placed on differentiating between erectile dysfunction and other sexual conditions, e.g. premature ejaculation. The nurse must encourage the patient to communicate openly, because the data collected will help to establish the severity and possible cause(s) of the problem. The following questions help to elicit appropriate responses from the patient:

1. **Tell me about the problems you are having with your erections?**
   Clarify what the exact nature of the problem is.
   Does the problem occur all of the time or only some of the time? (Intermittent erectile dysfunction may point to the problem being psychogenic in nature.)
   Do you experience early morning, nocturnal or spontaneous erections? (When the problem is psychogenic in nature, nocturnal and early morning erections are conserved.)
2. **Can you achieve an orgasm and are you still able to ejaculate?**
3. **Do you remember how the problem started?**
4. **How long has there been a problem?**
   If the onset is sudden, the origin of the problem is more likely to be psychogenic
   Gradual onset will point to an organic cause.
5. **What do you think is the cause of the problem?**
   The patient may have other concerns such as diabetes or cancer that he feels need to be dealt with.

Taking a sexual and general health history

A detailed history is the most important aspect of a holistic patient assessment. The primary aim of taking a history from the patient is to establish a diagnosis and to ensure that no important events that occurred in the past could have impinged on the current history (Guly, 1996). Once a careful history has been taken, this allows the nurse to plan appropriate therapeutic interventions and/or to refer to other healthcare agencies, and to provide key clues to the origin of the problem, understand perceptions, correct misconceptions, and ascertain concerns and expectations.

Details taken from the patient about his general health include checking for the following (Riley, 2001):

- Cardiovascular disease (including hypertension and peripheral vascular disease)
- Cardiovascular risk factors
- Depression
- Hypogonadism
- Hyperprolactinaemia
- Prostatic cancer (especially in men over 50 years of age)
- Therapeutic drugs known to have a propensity to impair erections
- Neurological disease
- Relationship issues
- Peyronie's disease
- Drug abuse
- Thyroid dysfunction.

The sexual health of the patient also needs to be investigated. The nurse needs to be considerate and to use tact and feel comfortable in him- or herself. If the nurse conveys discomfort, embarrassment or nervousness, the quality of data obtained will be of a poor standard. The interview should take place in a comfortable environment and privacy should be assured. It is acknowledged that nurses are busy practitioners. However, it is important to remember that this type of consultation demands more time than the general history-taking consultations, because often this type of consultation may present psychological barriers and is a very sensitive time for both the patient and the nurse. If appropriate, the patient should be encouraged to have his partner present at the consultation; however, this is not compulsory. Below is a list of some of the potential barriers that the nurse may encounter when taking a general and sexual health history.

Time

Discussing sexual health means that the nurse must manage the precious commodity of time in an effective manner in order to get as much from the consultation as possible.

Lack of knowledge

The nurse has a duty to ensure that his or her knowledge base about erectile dysfunction is up to date and correct. Misleading or giving wrong information to the patient is unacceptable. Nurses must be aware that the patient may also have a knowledge deficit.

Embarrassment

Discussing sexual health can be daunting for both the patient and the nurse. Taking the lead and being open and honest with the patient may reduce feelings of embarrassment.

Interruptions

Patients may fear that they can be overheard when discussing their intimate sexual health problems; the nurse must ensure that the possibility of being overheard is minimized. Ensure that telephones do not interrupt the consultation. Explain to the patient that what is said is said in confidence.

Before asking the man about his sexual health, the nurse must consider her or his personal feelings about sex and the language to use when talking about sexual issues. It is vital that the nurse refrain from making value judgements. Respect for the patient's sexual orientation or sexual preference must be paramount. There are no absolute rules about sexual health history taking, but the following points may be helpful:

- Be direct and ask straightforward questions – take a matter-of-fact approach.
- Use a vocabulary that the patient feels most comfortable with.
- Convey to the patient that you will not be judging him in any manner.
- Allow enough time for the consultation.
- Be aware of non-verbal communication.
- Summarize and check what the patient has said to you and allow him to correct any misconceptions that you may have.

To help the nurse to take a general and sexual health history competently a checklist is included in Table 5.1.

Summary of the recommendations for good history-taking practice

Nurses should be encouraged to take a general and sexual health history of patients who present with erectile dysfunction in order to assess the patient's needs in a holistic manner. It is vital that the nurse has an up-to-date knowledge base about erectile dysfunction. The nurse has several openings available for raising the issue of sexual health and erectile dysfunction. These occasions can be planned or opportunistic. The nurse should use effective communication skills, both verbally and non-verbally, to initiate and maintain the history-taking consultation. Appropriate vocabulary that is sensitive to the patient's needs is encouraged. The nurse must also be aware of other healthcare agencies that the patient can or may be referred to if appropriate.

Examination and investigations

Most patients require a limited physical assessment, e.g. the measurement of blood pressure and examination of the genitalia. When examining the genitalia, the nurse must focus on the penis, which must be examined carefully in order to identify any abnormalities such as micropenis, Peyronie's disease

Table 5.1 Checklist for taking a general sexual health history

Suggested strategies	Tick
A pleasant environment in which the consultation is to take place	
Privacy	
Freedom from interruptions (including telephones)	
Careful positioning of the furniture – spatial distancing	
Aim to provide a 'clinical'-free environment	
Ensure that you have adequate material resources available during the consultation	
Aim to provide a quiet environment	
Be aware of body language and the communication skills you are using	
Correct any ambiguities	
Respect the patient's choice of language, i.e. medical jargon or 'street talk'	
Focus on the patient's needs	
Speak directly – ask focused questions	
Employ sensitivity and empathy	
Empower the patient	
Accept that you may need to refer the patient to other healthcare agencies	
Avoid making any assumptions	
Do not judge or stereotype the patient	

Adapted from Jewitt (1995).

or hypospadias. Testicular size should be noted. To determine whether there is any peripheral vascular disease, the peripheral pulses must be palpated. To determine whether there are any associated neurological defects a neurological examination is needed, which should include assessment of perineal, penile and suprapubic sensation (Carson, 1999; Erectile Dysfunction Alliance, 1999). Further examination may be appropriate depending on the findings in the history, e.g. renal and endocrine system examination.

Laboratory investigations

As with the physical examination, the findings in the history (and the subsequent physical examination) may dictate what laboratory studies need to be undertaken. The laboratory studies help to detect any underlying undiagnosed metabolic conditions. All patients who have not previously been diagnosed with diabetes mellitus need to be tested to exclude it.

Serum analysis will include the following:

- Serum testosterone
- Plasma glucose measurement
- Creatinine and electrolytes
- Fasting lipids
- Luteinizing hormone
- Prolactin
- Liver function tests
- Haemoglobulinopathy screen (for African–Caribbean patients in order to exclude a sickling disorder – Erectile Dysfunction Alliance, 1999).

Carson (1999) discusses the value of using nocturnal penile tumescence monitoring to assess presence or absence of erectile function, its duration and rigidity. The presence or absence of nocturnal erections can help to differentiate neurogenic, psychogenic and vasculogenic causes of erectile dysfunction. The nocturnal penile tumescence monitor can be worn at night in the patient's own home.

Management options and choice of treatment

The management and treatment of erectile dysfunction over the past decade has changed considerably, moving from surgical intervention to injection therapy and oral medicines.

When a full assessment of the man's needs (and if appropriate his partner's) has been undertaken, expectations (which should be realistic) need to be stated and objectives set. At this stage the nurse can briefly explain to the patient what treatment options are available; one of them may be psychosexual therapy. The advantages of the various treatments available must be explained carefully to the patient, so that he is able to make an informed decision; this will mean that the nurse must have an up-to-date knowledge base. If the man decides that he wants to take the management of his erectile dysfunction no further, the nurse must respect this and reiterate that he or she will, if the patient so decides, discuss it further in the future.

Psychosexual therapy

Psychosexual therapy plays an important role in the management of erectile dysfunction and the use of an experienced psychosexual therapist is called for. The psychosexual therapist is a valuable member of the multidisciplinary approach to the management and treatment of erectile dysfunction.

Psychosexual therapists can offer the man (and his partner) support for the emotional difficulties associated with erectile dysfunction. Psychosexual therapy should not be overlooked in favour of the pharmacological and mechanical approaches available. Psychosexual therapy and other approaches to treatment can be undertaken concurrently rather than consecutively. Hartmann (1998) reviews the efficacy of psychosexual interventions and suggests that between 50 and 80 per cent of men report a positive outcome after attending psychosexual therapy.

It is important for the nurse to be aware of the effect erectile dysfunction can have, not only on the patient, but also on his partner. If the patient attends a consultation with his partner, the nurse must first ascertain that it is appropriate to discuss sexual problems with the partner present, because there may be underlying sexual issues that he may wish to keep to himself. There are advantages and disadvantages associated with psychosexual therapy (Erectile Dysfunction Alliance, 1999) (Table 5.2).

Table 5.2 The advantages and disadvantages of psychosexual therapy

Advantages	Disadvantages
• A physically non-invasive approach • Has the potential to involve the patient's partner if he so desires • Can lead to improvement in sexual function and satisfaction • May improve the couple's communication • Also addresses the partner's problems	• Patient and partner may be reluctant to attend • Service may not be available in every NHS locality • Time-consuming

Oral pharmacological agents

There are several oral treatments available for patients that are simple to use, non-invasive and with minimum side effects. The most common drug used today is sildenafil (Viagra). Sildenafil is a selective inhibitor of phosphodiesterase type 5 (PGE5). PGE5 is the main enzyme responsible for the breakdown of cyclic guanosine $3':5'$-monophosphate (cGMP); it acts by breaking down cGMP and helps to restore the erectile response in men. Some of the side effects associated with sildenafil are transient and mild, e.g. facial flushing, dyspepsia and slight headaches (Lobb-Rossini, 1999). Usually, sildenafil should be taken one hour before sexual activity; ingestion of a high fat meal will slow down its absorption. Patients who are using highly active antiretroviral therapy (HAART) must consult their HIV/AIDS practitioner before starting sildenafil. Sildenafil may react with certain antiretroviral drugs and therefore caution should be used before starting it (Camden and

Islington Community Health Service NHS Trust, 1998). A small study (Positive Treatment News, 2000) has found that indinavir (an antiretroviral drug) raised the levels of sildenafil, and it recommended that, when starting treatment with sildenafil, a smaller dose be given.

The advantages and disadvantages of sildenafil are shown in Table 5.3 (Erectile Dysfunction Alliance, 1999).

Table 5.3 The advantages and disadvantages of sildenafil

Advantages	Disadvantages
• Effective: 50–80% erectile improvement reported by users • Transient and mild side effects • Non-invasive	• Facilitates as opposed to initiates an erection • Contraindicated in patients who are taking nitrates, those with severe hepatic impairment, hypotension, hereditary degenerative retinal disorders, and recent cerebrovascular accident and myocardial infarction • Slower in onset compared with injected or transurethral treatments (e.g. transurethral alprostadil)

Intracavernosal prostaglandin

For those patients who are unable to take sildenafil, intracavernosal injection therapy may be of value. The use of intracavernosal injections has increased over the past decade and is the most common type of treatment. Wagner and Saenz de Tejada (1998) report response rates of 80 per cent with the use of intracavernosal injection therapy, but many men have a tendency to 'drop out' when using this type of treatment.

This particular type of treatment requires the patient to inject drugs, e.g. prostaglandin E_1 into the penis, which causes relaxation of the smooth muscle in the corpora cavernosa. Of men using this treatment, 40 per cent achieve an adequate erection that allows intercourse to take place. The nurse gives the initial injection and teaches the patient about the correct site to be used for injection. The patient can then, having been taught the correct procedure, administer it himself; however, he also requires ongoing monitoring of both technique and efficacy. Patients who have poor manual dexterity and poor eyesight may need their partners to be taught how to inject the penis. See Figure 5.5 for the correct method of injection.

There are few contraindications to the use of intracavernosal injection of vasoactive agents; however, it should not be given to men with haematological abnormalities such as sickle-cell anaemia, myeloma, leukaemia, and other coagulopathies or penile disorders.

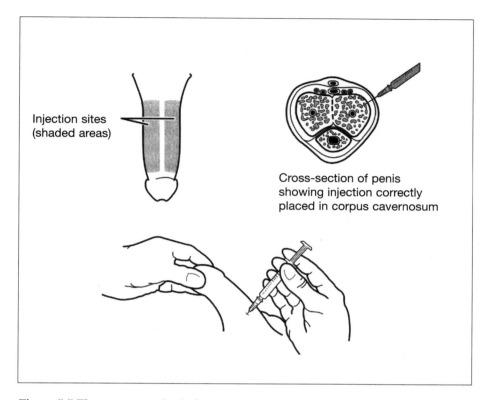

Injection sites (shaded areas)

Cross-section of penis showing injection correctly placed in corpus cavernosum

Figure 5.5 The correct method of injecting intracavernosal vasoactive agents. (Source: Nurse Education in Erectile Dysfunction (NEED). Pfizer Ltd., 2000.)

Peyronie's disease may occur if the patient is using intracavernosal injections, particularly if the injection site is not rotated. The cause of Peyronie's disease is unknown (Downey, 2000b). The disease is characterized by three features: penile pain, a lump in the flaccid penis and a deformity (a curve) in the erect penis. A hard plaque of fibrous tissue forms in the Buck's fascia or the septum between the corpora. Surgical intervention may be needed to correct the deformity.

As with other treatment modalities, there are associated advantages and disadvantages (Erectile Dysfunction Alliance, 1999) (Table 5.4).

Intraurethral delivery devices

This method of delivering the vasoactive agents for erection uses various devices that employ a non-injectable delivery system. The agent, in the form of a pellet containing synthesized prostaglandin E_1, is administered directly into the urethra. The prostaglandin is quickly absorbed into the corpus spongiosum and the corpora cavernosa; this increased blood flow to the corpora

Table 5.4 The advantages and disadvantages of intracavernosal prostaglandin

Advantages	Disadvantages
• Effective in providing men with erections adequate for intercourse • Few contraindications or interactions, therefore suitable for a wide range of patients • Rapid onset • Has demonstrated recovery of spontaneous erection in some patients	• Mild penile pain on injection • Penile fibrosis, bleeding and bruising • Patient education is needed • May be problematic for patients with poor manual dexterity and poor eyesight • Low risk of priapism

cavernosa promotes an erection within approximately 5–10 minutes and can last for up to one hour. Patients who choose this type of treatment need information on how to use the non-injectable delivery system (Figure 5.6).

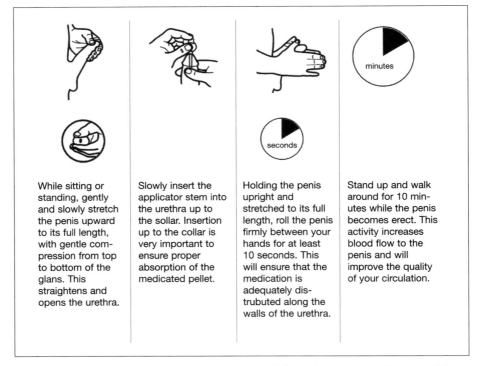

While sitting or standing, gently and slowly stretch the penis upward to its full length, with gentle compression from top to bottom of the glans. This straightens and opens the urethra.

Slowly insert the applicator stem into the urethra up to the sollar. Insertion up to the collar is very important to ensure proper absorption of the medicated pellet.

Holding the penis upright and stretched to its full length, roll the penis firmly between your hands for at least 10 seconds. This will ensure that the medication is adequately distrubuted along the walls of the urethra.

Stand up and walk around for 10 minutes while the penis becomes erect. This activity increases blood flow to the penis and will improve the quality of your circulation.

Figure 5.6 Transurethral drug administration and the information patients need for successful and effective use of the device. (Source: Nurse Education in Erectile Dysfunction (NEED). Pfizer Ltd., 2000.)

The advantages and disadvantages associated with intraurethral delivery are shown in Table 5.5 (Erectile Dysfunction Alliance, 1999).

Table 5.5 The advantages and disadvantages of of intraurethral delivery devices

Advantages	Disadvantages
• Suitable for a wide range of patients, including those with a fear of needles (needle phobia) • Proven to provide an adequate erection for intercourse	• Some debate about efficacy • May cause discomfort in lower limb varicosities; requires good dexterity, eyesight and has to be administered post-micturition • Slower acting than injection • Penile urethral discomfort • Patients need educating to use the device effectively • Partner may complain of vaginal irritation

Mechanical devices: vacuum constriction devices

Lewis and Witherington (1997) state that the overall clinical success rate associated with the use of vacuum constriction devices is quoted at approximately 90 per cent. Mechanical devices are the simplest and the least expensive treatment (Wagner and Saenz de Tejada, 1998). The device works by aspirating blood into the penis via a vacuum tube placed around it, resulting in engorgement of the corpus cavernosum and therefore relaxation of the smooth muscle. The pump is activated by hand or can be battery controlled. The blood remains in the corpus cavernosum through the use of a restricting band placed over the base of the penis; this maintains venous stasis without decreased arterial inflow.

External vacuum device

After approximately 30 minutes with the constriction band on the base of the penis, the patient may find it uncomfortable and oedema may occur; if this happens the restriction band should be removed (Figure 5.7). There are relatively few side effects and contraindications associated with the use of a vacuum device. However, patients with haematological abnormalities, e.g. those on anticoagulation therapy, or patients with leukaemia or sickle-cell disease, should not use the device. There are associated complications with the use of such devices, e.g. plaque formation and Peyronie's disease.

The advantages and disadvantages of this type of treatment are shown in Table 5.6 (Erectile Dysfunction Alliance, 1999).

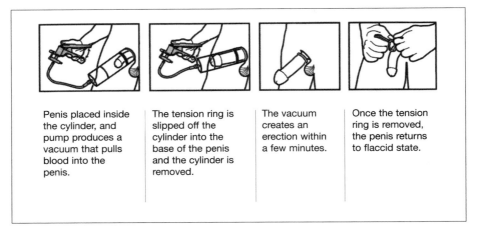

| Penis placed inside the cylinder, and pump produces a vacuum that pulls blood into the penis. | The tension ring is slipped off the cylinder into the base of the penis and the cylinder is removed. | The vacuum creates an erection within a few minutes. | Once the tension ring is removed, the penis returns to flaccid state. |

Figure 5.7 External vacuum constriction device. (Source: Nurse Education in Erectile Dysfunction (NEED). Pfizer Ltd., 2000.)

Table 5.6 The advantages and disadvantages of vacuum constriction devices

Advantages	Disadvantages
• Low incidence of side effects • Suitable for a wide range of patients • Can be used long term	• Contraindicated in patients with bleeding disorders • Can be seen as cumbersome • Temperature changes (penis may feel cold) • Sensation of ejaculation may be impaired

Penile prosthesis and surgical intervention

When other treatments are unsuccessful or cannot be used because of contraindications, surgical intervention may be the last resort.

Arterial revascularization (arterial reconstructive surgery) may be undertaken in those men who have evidence of arterial occlusive disease. The inferior epigastric artery is microscopically anastomosed by an end-to-end or end-to-side anastomosis with the deep dorsal artery of the penis. Using this technique blood is redirected from the inferior epigastric artery to the central cavernosal arteries. In those patients who are carefully selected, this may have a success rate of up to 65 per cent (Goldstein, 1996). Those patients with significant atherosclerosis or atherosclerotic risk factors should not be considered for such surgical intervention.

For those men with veno-occlusive disease, venous surgery with extensive ligation of the veins that drain the corpora cavernosa is often the last resort before penile implantation is considered (Wagner and Saenz de Tejada, 1998). The outcome of such surgery has poor results (Carson, 1999).

Prosthetic penile implants

There are many types of penile implant available; these implants provide penile rigidity and are classified as semi-rigid or inflatable. Steege et al. (1986) suggest that the implants provide satisfactory penile rigidity, normal sensation, erectile size and excellent partner/patient satisfaction. The various types of surgical implants can be seen in Figure 5.8.

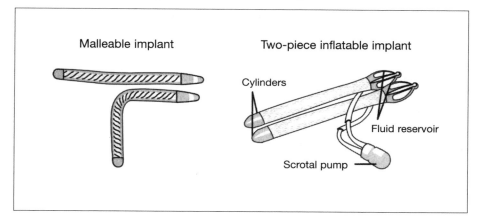

Figure 5.8 Various prostheses to produce penile erection. (Source: Nurse Education in Erectile Dysfunction (NEED). Pfizer Ltd., 2000.)

The pump and reservoir are placed in the scrotum when the two-piece inflatable prosthesis is used; they are used to inflate the cylinders into the erect position. The cylinders are deflated by pressing a valve at the base of the pump, returning the fluid to the reservoir. In a three-piece inflatable prosthesis, only the pump is in the scrotum, the reservoir being in the abdominal cavity. Semi-rigid and malleable implants can be implanted into the penis to provide penile erection.

Pre- and postoperative care of the patient with penile implants

Infection is a major potential complication of penile implants and can occur in up to 3–5 per cent of patients, so preparations are made preoperatively to reduce this risk. As a result of this, Carson (1999) recommends that, for surgical intervention, as a prophylactic measure, the patient commences antibiotic therapy 1 hour before surgery and continues to take antibiotics for at least 72 hours postoperatively. Some surgeons require patients to have preoperative povidone–iodine or chlorhexidine baths. The patient should be given enough time to express his fears and worries, and the nurse should offer him support and comfort. Advice needs to be given to the patient about the type of implant and how to inflate and deflate it; it may help to show the patient the different types of implant. Referral may need to be made to a psychosexual therapist.

To reduce the effects of oedema, the patient should be encouraged to use ice packs on the genitalia, and the penis should be elevated with a scrotal support or supportive underpants. Regular analgesics should be offered, with the aim of ensuring that the patient is pain free. The wound should be observed for signs of breakdown and haemorrhage, and the patient's pulse, blood pressure and temperature need to be monitored on a regular basis to identify any potential problems. It is important that the patient's ability to pass urine is documented; the nurse may need to support the patient to urinate. If the patient is unable to pass urine, the surgeon must be informed, because catheterization may be needed.

A potential problem with the implanted device may occur, and this could be displacement of the parts of the device or a device malfunction. The patient must be informed that he should return to the ward immediately if he experiences any problems after discharge. Inflation of the device should not occur until 4–6 weeks after surgery. There are several advantages and disadvantages associated with surgical intervention and penile implants (Erectile Dysfunction Alliance, 1999) (Table 5.7).

Table 5.7 The advantages and disadvantages of surgical intervention and penile implants

Advantages	Disadvantages
• Long-term use; negates the use of injection and oral medication or when other forms of treatment are contraindicated • Of value in patients with penile fibrosis	• An invasive operative procedure; infection is a possibility postoperatively • The prosthesis (semi-rigid and malleable prosthesis) may protrude under clothing • Mechanical problems are reported with the device • Pain and oedema

When the correct management approach has been agreed with the patient (and if appropriate, his partner), a system for following the patient up must be planned. Follow-up is important to assess patient satisfaction (audit), to monitor side effects of treatment and to assess efficacy of treatment. The Erectile Dysfunction Alliance (1999) suggests a review point between four weeks and six months; this allows for a change or cessation of treatment if appropriate. For patients who are being treated with intracavernosal injections, long-term follow-up is vital in order to detect penile fibrosis.

Conclusion

Erectile dysfunction is a common sexual health problem that affects a signifi-cant number of men and their partners in the UK. The number of men with the disorder is difficult to estimate for a variety of reasons, e.g. men often feel too embarrassed to seek healthcare advice in order to address this distress-ing condition. Perring and Moran (1995) report that patients frequently feel that they are failures; they are often devastated and have profound feelings of humiliation.

Nurses must remember that erectile dysfunction is a not a disease; it is a symptom of an underlying pathology that can be either organic or psy-chogenic in nature. The condition can impinge on a man's self-esteem, his social life and his relationship with his partner. Often men are reluctant to seek advice despite the fact that there are effective, safe and easy-to-use treat-ments available.

Men must be encouraged in the primary healthcare setting to seek help and advice from the practice nurse or the GP as soon as they begin to ex-perience any problems. Riley (2001) states that any delay in seeking help and advice for erectile dysfunction can be costly. The nurse plays an impor-tant and active role in encouraging men to come forward and seek assistance. Early interested interventions are vital if the man is to feel that the nurse and the other members of the healthcare team are to take his complaint seriously.

The nurse needs to have an in-depth knowledge base about the condition, to devote sufficient time for the man to talk about his problems and, most importantly, to address his or her own attitudes and how comfortable he or she feels talking about intimate sexual issues with the patient. There are national and local guidelines available to nurses that may help to provide the patient with the most appropriate care he needs.

It is vital that an in-depth assessment of the patient is undertaken in order to identify any abnormalities that may contribute to the development of erec-tile dysfunction. A comprehensive assessment may reveal the presence of a treatable medical condition which, if not identified, could put the patient's life at risk.

For men to make an informed decision about treatment of the condition, they must know what treatment options are available and what the advan-tages and disadvantages of the various treatments are. Nurses must have this information available and be prepared to impart it in a manner that the patient finds acceptable. The role of the nurse as advocate is central to the successful treatment of this distressing condition, which a significant num-ber of men will face.

There are many treatments available for men to choose from; the ideal treatment is yet to be found, but technology has allowed many innovative and important advances to be made. Government thinking needs to be convinced that erectile dysfunction is a serious condition, and that men who have it are entitled to effective treatment on the NHS despite the current costs of treatment. Although the recent Government's decision to allow vacuum devices to be prescribable under the NHS is a welcome move, more influence is needed to ensure that the Government remove some of the inequalities in legislation for erectile dysfunction.

Nurses can encourage more debate and discussion about erectile dysfunction by ensuring that there is a greater openness about the subject, which may make it easier for men to come forward and discuss their problems. Nurse educationalists should address the complex issue of sexual health at all levels of the educational system, i.e. nurse education pre- and post-registration.

CHAPTER SIX

Prostatic disease

Prostate disease is now receiving more attention than it has in the past. Prostate cancer is a puzzling disease insofar as it is impossible to differentiate between slow-growing tumours that cause no harm and fast-growing (aggressive) tumours that can kill if not treated early enough. The Department of Health (2000c) has concluded that more needs to be done to detect prostate cancer and to improve the treatment and care of men diagnosed with it. Plans to introduce a Prostate Cancer Risk Management Programme by the Government, along with current initiatives such as *The NHS Plan* (Department of Health, 2000a) and *The NHS Cancer Plan* (Department of Health, 2000b), can only help nurses to provide men with quality care and treatment.

This chapter focuses on two specific prostatic diseases:

1. Benign prostatic hyperplasia (BPH)
2. Prostate cancer.

For a full understanding of how prostatic disease affects the sexual health of men, nurses must have an in-depth understanding of the prostate gland, its anatomy and physiology, as well as its role and function in male reproduction.

In the USA, prostate cancer is the most commonly diagnosed cancer in men; there were an estimated 198 000 new cases in 2001 (Greenlee et al., 2001). In the UK and the European Union, this cancer is the second most common cancer in men (lung cancer is the most common male cancer). In 1997, there were over 20 000 new cases in the UK and an estimated 134 000 new cases in 1996 in the EU (Cancer Research Campaign, 2001).

Anatomy and physiology

The prostate gland is relatively small in size, weighs approximately 20 g, is doughnut shaped and the size of a chestnut, and is usually about 4 cm in diameter. The word prostate is derived from the ancient Greek language: *pro* meaning in front of and *statos* meaning standing. The prostate gland in the male human surrounds the urethra, protecting the exit to the bladder. Its position here may account for the small numbers of young men who present with urinary tract infection, because the prostate gland has antibacterial properties (Kirby and Kirby, 1999). The prostate gland surrounds the superior aspect of the urethra and is situated inferior to the urinary bladder. The gland is embedded in fibromuscular tissue (Robinson and Huether, 1998).

The prostate has three separate zones: the central zone, the peripheral zone and the transitional zone which lies between them. These zones are susceptible to specific types of prostatic disease. A common site for the development of prostate cancer is the peripheral zone; the transitional zone is where the adenomatous nodules form, which are associated with BPH (Kirby and Kirby, 1999). Glandular tissue can be found in the outer zone (this is the lateral and posterior portion of the prostate gland) and the inner zone (nearest to the urethra) is made up of mucous glands. Fillingham and Douglas (1997a) point out that there are no truly defined zones within the prostate gland, but for clinical purposes specific areas are identified within the gland using this categorization.

The prostate gland is made up of a network of secretory tubules. Contractile smooth muscle fibres surround every tubule; the gland itself is supported by connective tissue. During ejaculation, the prostate gland contracts rhythmically and secretes prostatic fluid as semen moves through the prostatic portion of the urethra; this prostatic fluid is mixed with the semen. The neck of the bladder contracts in order to prevent retrograde ejaculation. Prostatic fluid empties via the prostatic ducts into the urethra. The milky prostatic fluid contributes to approximately 20 per cent of the ejaculate. The fluid has a slightly alkaline pH, which helps sperm to survive in the acid environment of the woman's reproductive tract (Robinson and Huether, 1998). The fluid contains a small amount of citric acid, some lipids and a few enzymes. The reason for prostatic fluid's alkalinity is that it contains a significant number of bicarbonate ions (Creager, 1983).

Prostatic secretions contain high concentrations of prostate-specific antigen (PSA). PSA is a single-chain glycoprotein consisting of 93 per cent amino acids and 7 per cent carbohydrate. Functionally, it is a kallikrein-like protease secreted by the epithelial cells lining the acini and ducts of the prostate gland. This strong protease liquefies semen after ejaculation by breaking down the protein seminogelin and, it is believed, promotes the motility of sperm so that they can travel through the female reproductive tract.

Circulating testicular hormones, in adequate amounts, are needed for the secretory function of the prostate gland. Growth of the gland and the secretory function are closely linked to changes in plasma concentrations of the circulating testicular hormones.

From birth to puberty the prostate gland increases slowly in size; after puberty it increases rapidly in size up until about the age of 30. Stability in growth remains until about 45 years of age, when the gland enlarges further; it is at this stage that abnormalities begin to develop and the patient may present symptomatically or asymptomatically.

Benign prostatic hyperplasia

In most men aged over 40 years the transitional zone of the prostate gland starts to show signs of hyperplasia. One in 10 men presents with urinary out-flow obstruction that results from enlargement of the gland. BPH is the most prevalent disorder aggravating the prostate. Downey (2000a) estimates that there are over 2.5 million men in the UK who have lower urinary tract symptoms caused by BPH.

The aetiology of BPH is unknown. Testicular sex hormones such as testosterone and androgens appear to play an active part in cell division through diffusion and conversion of the testicular sex hormones by certain enzymes, e.g. 5α-reductase. The usual balance with cell death is interrupted and BPH results. Growth factors activated by cell division cause epidermal growth and enlargement of the prostate gland may occur. Interestingly, BPH is unknown in eunuchs (Kumar and Clark, 1996).

Bott and Kirby (2002) suggest that when considering BPH it may be help-ful also to consider clinical BPH as coexisting with benign prostatic enlargement or lower urinary tract symptoms. BPH is rarely life threatening, but often it can have a detrimental effect on a patient's life and those he is closest to.

Signs and symptoms

In most patients the onset of BPH is slow, the extent and severity of the signs and symptoms depending on how long the prostate gland has been enlarged. As a patient with BPH ages, the severity increases. There are several signs and symptoms with which the patient may present:

- An increase in frequency of micturition – up to 12 times per day.
- Nocturia – may get up several times in the night to urinate.
- Urinary tract infection – a result of the bladder not fully emptying.
- Hesitancy – delay occurring when the patient wishes to pass urine.
- Dysuria – pain on passing urine as a result of infection.
- Chronic retention of urine with overflow – may be confused with incontinence.
- Acute retention of urine – distended bladder and severe abdominal pain.

As the prostate expands, this often brings with it long-term prostatic outflow obstruction and, because of this, other secondary events can arise. The bladder, in response to outflow obstruction, initially enlarges and thickens; flow rate and emptying of the bladder are normal at this stage. However, as time passes, the detrusor muscle weakens and the bladder stretches, becomes ineffective and fails to empty completely, resulting in an atonic bladder. The residual urine in the bladder has the potential to become infected easily. With worsening back flow, bladder diverticula can occur; the ureters may dilate as a result of the back pressure, hydronephrosis can ensue and renal failure becomes an extreme possibility (Fillingham and Douglas, 1997a; Downey, 2000a). When these symptoms are prolonged, there may be a necessity for prostatic surgery (Arrhigi et al., 1990).

If left untreated, the slow progression of BPH and worsening of the associated symptoms affect the patient's quality of life, and his ability to carry out normal activities deteriorates; eventually acute retention of urine ensues. The patient is often prevented from enjoying outdoor activities, and he has to restrict use of his own or public transport. He may need to restrict his fluid intake in the evenings to reduce the number of times he has to get up to urinate in the night. His social life may deteriorate and he can become socially isolated; the increased number of times he needs to pass urine can also have an effect on his sexual life.

Making a diagnosis

Making a diagnosis of BPH is complex. A detailed and in-depth history from the patient reveals many rich data for making the diagnosis. Lower urinary tract symptoms (associated with BPH) are common as a result of the growing prostate gland. To make a distinct diagnosis of BPH, other pathologies have to be excluded. Bott and Kirby (2000) suggest that these other pathologies can also be closely related to lower urinary tract symptoms:

- Malignancy:
  - prostate cancer
  - carcinoma *in situ* (e.g. cancer of the bladder)
- Infection:
  - bacterial
  - tuberculosis
- Neurological:
  - Parkinson's disease
  - cerebrovascular event
  - multiple sclerosis
- Mechanical:
  - urethral stricture
  - severe phimosis

- Drug induced:
  - antidepressants
  - anticholinergics
  - diuretics.

Most clinicians, according to Kirby and Kirby (1999), ask the patient three questions:

1. Do you wake up at night to pass urine?
2. Is your urinary flow reduced?
3. Are you bothered by your bladder symptoms?

If the response to any of the questions is positive, then an attempt to quantify the severity of the patient's symptoms should be undertaken by issuing the patient with a self-administered questionnaire – the International Prostate Symptoms Score (IPSS). This well-validated tool asks the patient to give a score to the following symptoms:

- Incomplete bladder emptying
- Frequency
- Intermittency
- Urgency
- Weak stream
- Straining
- Nocturia.

What the IPSS does not do, however, is predict the extent of outlet obstruction. The IPSS can be used to gain a baseline for the patient's symptoms and also to assess the efficacy of any subsequent treatment (see Downey, 2000a, for further details of the IPSS).

Investigations

As well as taking a detailed history and assessing the IPSS, a physical examination is needed. Palpation of the abdomen may reveal a distended abdomen, a result of chronic or acute urinary retention or other abnormal intra-abdominal pathology. A digital rectal examination should be performed because this may uncover the coexistence of prostate cancer and also provides an indication of prostate size. The consistency of a 'normal prostate gland' on palpation is said to have the same consistency as the tip of the nose. Assessment of urinary flow rate can help establish whether there are problems with urinary stream. If there is a suspicion of urinary tract infection, a mid-stream specimen of urine needs to be collected and analysed by microscopy, culture and sensitivity. In those patients with excessive frequency of micturition and dysuria, it may be prudent to perform urine cytology to determine whether there is any evidence of bladder carcinoma.

A non-invasive assessment of bladder function using urodynamic measurements is often indicated, and this may also be performed by ultrasonography. An intravenous urogram can determine whether there is any impairment of the urinary tract as a result of outflow obstruction. Kirby and Kirby (1999) state that a mandatory cystourethroscopy is needed if there is a history of haematuria or any suspicion of carcinoma of the bladder.

Various blood samples are taken. In men with BPH, serum creatinine is elevated, so blood should be taken to measure this; renal function tests are also indicated. Kirby and Kirby (1999) state that the measurement of PSA in men suspected of having BPH is controversial. A full blood count is also needed.

If the patient is experiencing any sexual difficulties, it may be appropriate to refer him to a psychosexual therapist. This will allow him to express any anxieties that he may have currently or in the future. He may wish to have his partner present at the consultation and his desire to do so, or not, must be respected.

Treatment options

When the definitive diagnosis of BPH has been made, the treatment depends on the severity of the patient's symptoms as measured by the IPSS, flow rate and amount of residual urine in the bladder, the presence of co-morbidity, and discussion with the patient about his choice.

Downey (2000a) and Bott and Kirby (2002) use the term 'watchful waiting'. 'Watchful waiting' is implicated when the patient is not troubled with his symptoms and there is no evidence of bladder stones, recurrent urinary tract infections and impairment of renal function. Regular monitoring of the patient's condition is needed and he should be recalled on a frequent basis to give a history of his health, have his urinary peak flow measured and make a self-assessment using the IPSS.

Generally speaking the most popular form of treatment for BPH is surgical intervention – transurethral resection of the prostate gland (TURP). Indeed, Kirby and Kirby (1999) state that, for those patients with the following complications of BPH, TURP is the standard therapy:

• Acute or chronic retention of urine
• Bladder stones
• Upper tract dilatation
• Recurrent urinary tract infections
• Haematuria.

For those uncomplicated cases, the most appropriate form of therapy is medical treatment. Medical treatment is in fact the first line of treatment; surgery is considered in those men who do not respond to medical treatment, or whose disease progresses despite drug therapy.

Pharmacological therapies

There are two main pharmacological agents that are considered for men with BPH:

1. α-Adrenergic blockers, e.g. doxazosin, prazosin and terazosin
2. 5α-Reductase type II inhibitors, e.g. finasteride.

The α-adrenergic blockers act by inhibiting the smooth muscle contractions in the prostate, prostatic urethra and bladder neck; this action facilitates voiding. Finasteride is a competitive inhibitor of 5α-reductase, which is the enzyme responsible for the conversion of testosterone to dihydrotestosterone. This androgen is primarily responsible for prostatic growth and enlargement; as a result of the action of finasteride prostatic volume decreases and urine outflow increases. The patient should be aware that, as 5α-reductase is found in the hair follicle of the scalp, some patients may detect a reversal of the male balding pattern. As finasteride is excreted in the semen, it is advisable that, if the man's sexual partner is pregnant, condoms be used. Men should be warned that there might be a reduced amount of ejaculate if taking finasteride.

The nurse must be aware (and educate the patient) that those patients who are taking some α-adrenergic blockers are at risk of postural hypotension and syncope. Elderly patients may be prone to falling, so the first dose should be taken when the patient goes to bed. The nurse should encourage the patient to sit or lie down if he feels dizzy, or if he is sweating or feeling fatigued, and to get up only when these symptoms abate completely. In addition, the nurse should encourage the patient to stand up or get out of bed slowly to prevent postural hypotension.

Surgical intervention for BPH

Surgical excision of the adenomatous tissue that forms on the transitional zone of the prostatic urethra has remarkable effects on the symptoms and the quality of the patient's urinary outflow. A consequence of this means that there is also a reduction in the amount of residual urine.

As a result of the advances and the success of medical interventions discussed earlier, over the past 15 years the number of men requiring surgical intervention has halved (Bott and Kirby, 2002). Just as advances have been made with medical therapies, surgical techniques have also improved and become more refined, e.g. the advent of laser, microwave and thermotherapy.

However, surgical intervention is not without side effects. Mebust et al. (1989) suggest that where surgical intervention is undertaken complications arise in approximately 18 per cent of cases, with a small but significant mortality. Some of the complications have a significant and direct effect on the man's sexual health. Over 50 per cent of those men who undergo TURP experience retrograde ejaculation, because removal of the prostate tissue at the bladder neck may cause the seminal fluid to flow backwards into the urinary bladder, as opposed to forwards through the urethra during ejaculation. A smaller percentage of men develop erectile dysfunction (Smeltzer and Bare, 2000). As a result of this, Kirby and Kirby (1999) suggest that surgical intervention should be confined to those men with absolute indications for surgery, i.e. bladder stones or persistent haematuria, as a result of BPH, or in those men for whom pharmacological intervention has been unsuccessful.

There are several treatment options available to a man needing prostatic surgery. The interventions currently available are becoming 'less invasive', e.g. laser, transurethral microwave therapy and electrovaporization. It is the size of the prostate gland, a large gland weighing over 60 g, that is more likely to require an open approach to remove it. The choice of surgical intervention, the age of the patient, the severity of the obstruction, the condition of the patient and the presence of associated diseases depend on the approach to be taken.

Transurethral resection of the prostate gland
TURP is the most common type of surgical procedure performed for BPH. A resectoscope is passed via the urethra with a loop for cutting, diathermy and an optical source; the transurethral approach is a closed procedure. As the electrical loop chips away at the gland the diathermy controls the bleeding. Nurses need to be aware of the advantages and disadvantages of the various surgical approaches in order to impart this information to their patients (Table 6.1).

Specific preoperative nursing care
An in-depth assessment of the patient preoperatively is vital in order to ascertain the state of the patient's general health. A full explanation of the proposed surgery must be clearly given to the patient so that he can make an informed choice about the surgery. The patient may need an explanation of where the prostate gland is situated and its functions. The nurse must remember that the patient may be reluctant to discuss his condition, because it will impinge on his sexuality. Furthermore, it is related to his genitalia; as a result of this the nurse must ensure privacy and adopt a sensitive approach

Table 6.1 Advantages and disadvantages of transurethral resection of the prostate gland (TURP)

Advantages	Disadvantages	Nursing implications
• Avoids an abdominal incision (no abdominal scarring) • Safer for those patients who may be a 'surgical risk' • Shorter periods of time spent in hospital and a faster recovery rate • Lower morbidity rates • Less pain	• Requires a highly skilled surgeon, i.e. the surgeon must be careful not to damage the external sphincter at the base of the bladder as this may result in incontinence • Recurrent obstruction (caused by prostate tissue growing back), urethral trauma and stricture formation • Delayed bleeding may occur; monitor haemorrhage	• Monitor fluid balance; prevent fluid overload • Control pain • Observe for symptoms of urethral stricture, i.e. dysuria, straining, weak urinary stream

to the proposed surgery and potential complications that may arise. It is important that the nurse explains the possibility of postoperative retrograde ejaculation. This aspect of the patient's sexual health can often be overlooked or ignored, or it can be taken for granted that other healthcare professionals, such as the doctor, will deal with the issue. The nurse provides information for the patient in a language that he understands; she or he must also inform the patient about the postoperative period and the type of urinary drainage system that he will have *in situ*.

Specific postoperative care
The major postoperative goals for the patient include correction of fluid balance, relief of pain and discomfort, and prevention of infection; catheter blockage and monitoring of haemorrhage are also dealt with. Other complications following TURP include deep vein thrombosis and pulmonary embolism.

The management of the patient's pain is of paramount importance and prescribed analgesia must be given and its effects monitored to assess efficacy. Bladder spasms may occur after TURP and prescribed medication to relax smooth muscle can help relieve the spasms, which are caused by the pressure exerted by the inflated balloon on the bladder wall around the trigone.

Despite the intraoperative use of diathermy, the prostate gland is a highly vascular gland; bleeding and haemorrhage may occur and careful monitoring of the patient is needed. Blood pressure and pulse should be measured every 15 minutes and the frequency reduced as the patient's condition dictates.

When the patient returns from the operating theatre, he will have bladder irrigation running via a three-way catheter; prescribed fluids such as intravenous 0.1% saline are used to irrigate the bladder. Urinary output at this stage is expected to be bright red; however, if this continues, the doctor must be informed because this may indicate a haemorrhage. The irrigation should be titrated to the colour of the urinary outflow, e.g. dark red outflow – the speed of the irrigation should be increased; and pink (rose) outflow – the irrigation can be slowed down. The aim is to provide enough irrigation to prevent the formation of clots, which can lead to obstruction of the urethral catheter. If the catheter does become blocked, the patient complains of pain and the need to pass urine, and his abdomen may be distended; in this case a bladder washout may be needed.

The amount of bladder irrigation must be carefully monitored and the nurse has to ensure that the total output exceeds the input. It is vital that documentation on a fluid balance chart is up to date, correct and in line with the UKCC's (1998) standards for documentation. If the irrigation fluid is being absorbed into the bloodstream as a result of extravasation, the transurethral syndrome can occur. If this happens, it is an emergency and so the nurse must vigilant at all times. As the irrigation fluid is absorbed into the bloodstream, the blood becomes diluted and circulatory overload occurs. The patient may become confused and disoriented; he may have a seizure as a result of low plasma sodium and cardiac arrest may ensue. Irrigation fluid must be stopped immediately and intravenous fluids slowed down.

To detect infection, the patient must have his temperature recorded every four hours (or more frequently depending on the patient's condition); the use of a rectal thermometer to record temperature must be avoided. The patient may have been prescribed antibiotics if a urinary tract infection was or is suspected. If symptoms persist, a catheter specimen may be needed to determine the infective agent and to treat it with the most appropriate antibiotic therapy. To reduce the risk of infection, a closed urine drainage system must be used and maintained. If the system needs to be broken, e.g. to perform a bladder washout, this must be done using a strict aseptic technique. The insertion site of the catheter is kept clean by using soap and water.

On discharge, the patient should have an outpatient appointment made for about six weeks after surgery. The nurse should encourage the patient to rest and avoid any heavy lifting and straining at defecation (the Valsalva effect). If the patient works, it is usual for him to have 4–5 weeks off. Fillingham and Douglas (1997a) recommend that the nurse should warn the patient that, about two weeks after surgery, he might experience urethral bleeding. This, the patient should be told, is normal because it is a result of 'encrustations' falling off during the healing process. The patient should increase his oral fluid intake and report the incident to his GP if it does not abate. Sexual intercourse (including masturbation) should be refrained from for at least two weeks.

Should the patient suffer with dysuria, fever, urgency or frequency, he should visit his GP because this may be caused by urinary tract infection.

Other approaches to prostatectomy

Suprapubic prostatectomy
This procedure involves removing the prostate gland through an abdominal incision. The advantage of this approach is that it allows removal of a gland of any size. The disadvantages associated with the suprapubic approach are shown in Table 6.2.

Table 6.2 Advantages and disadvantages of suprapubic prostatectomy

Advantages	Disadvantages	Nursing implications
• Offers a wider area of exploration	• Requires a surgical incision through the bladder	• Close monitoring of the patient's condition for shock and haemorrhage
• Allows for examination of cancerous lymph nodes	• May be difficult to control haemorrhage	• Ensure meticulous aseptic technique when dealing with and around the suprapubic incision site
• Surgeon can completely remove the obstructing gland	• Leakage of urine around the suprapubic tubing	
• Allows treatment of associated bladder lesions	• Prolonged and more uncomfortable recovery	• Control pain

Perineal prostatectomy
To remove the prostate gland, the incision is made in the perineum. It is often used when other approaches are unsuitable and it also facilitates open biopsy. The complications associated with this particular approach are shown in Table 6.3.

Table 6.3 Advantages and disadvantages of perineal prostatectomy

Advantages	Disadvantages	Nursing implications
• Provides a direct anatomical approach	• Higher incidence of urinary incontinence and impotence	• Must not use rectal thermometer, enema and rectal tubing after surgery
• Permits gravitational drainage	• Potential damage to rectum and external sphincter	
• Very effective for radical cancer therapy	• Restricted operative field	• Patient will need to be provided with a foam-rubber ring to sit on
• Low mortality rate		
• Lower incidences of shock	• Higher incidence of infection (as a result of incisional site being close to rectum)	• Ensure that perianal care is meticulous
• Ideal for very old patients and those deemed at 'surgical risk'		• Control pain

Retropubic prostatectomy

This approach is more common than the suprapubic approach. The incision is made in the low abdomen and the prostate gland is approached between the symphysis pubis and the bladder. There is no entry into the bladder. This approach is suitable for larger prostate glands (Table 6.4).

Table 6.4 Advantages and disadvantages of retropubic prostatectomy

Advantages	Disadvantages	Nursing implications
• There is no incision made into the urinary bladder • Allows the surgeon to see and control any bleeding • Shorter recovery period • Less damage to the bladder sphincter	• Unable to treat associated bladder disease • An increased likelihood of haemorrhage	• Close observation for signs of haemorrhage • Control pain

Transurethral incision of the prostate (TUIP)

This approach is indicated when the prostate gland is small, i.e. less than 30 g, and is becoming a more popular choice of treatment in the UK. One or two incisions are made into the prostate gland via the urethra in order to reduce the pressure of the prostate gland on the urethra. This procedure may be performed as a day case under general or local anaesthetic (Table 6.5).

Table 6.5 Advantages and disadvantages of transurethral incision of the prostate (TUIP)

Advantages	Disadvantages	Nursing implications
• Similar results to TURP • No bladder neck contracture • Reduced cases of erectile dysfunction induced by the procedure • Lower incidence of retrograde ejaculation	• The surgeon must be highly skilled • Recurrent obstruction • Higher incidence of urethral trauma	• Monitor for haemorrhage • Control • Day-care admission with associated preparation and discharge information

Transurethral needle abliteration (TUNA)

This approach is relatively new and recent innovations such as TUNA need to be assessed to determine whether they are as effective as TURP. The procedure is performed by inserting a needle into the prostate and applying very-high-frequency radiowaves. The patient can be treated as a day case. In some instances the patient may need to have a urinary catheter inserted after the procedure. The nurse must advise the patient about the management of the catheter when he goes home and inform him of follow-up arrangements, i.e. outpatient appointments.

Prostactic stent insertion

A prostatic stent made of either macroporous tubular mesh or a coiled metal spring is inserted into the urethra; a cystoscope and transrectal ultrasonography are then used to advance the stent into the prostatic urethra. The patient is prescribed prophylactic antibiotic therapy to reduce the incidence of infection resulting from the presence of the stent. The nurse must be aware of the fact that the stent sits in the prostatic urethra and on no account should a urethral catheter be passed; if catheterization is needed, this will be suprapubic in nature. For this reason, patients should be encouraged to carry a card with them pointing out that they are using a prostatic stent.

The number of cases of BPH continues to rise as the population generally ages. In the past, the most common approach to the treatment of BPH has been 'watchful waiting' and surgical intervention. There are more advances being made in the medical management of the condition, and a move to treat patients less invasively means that the number of open prostatectomies has decreased. According to Bott and Kirby (2002), such an increase in choice of treatment means that the patient and the clinician are able to tailor the treatment to the needs of the individual. Nurses have a central role to play, by providing the patient with information that allows him to make a decision that is truly informed and based on sound fact.

Cancer of the prostate

Incidence

In 2000, worldwide, there were over 543 000 cases of prostate cancer with over 204 000 deaths annually. There has been an annual increase worldwide of 1.7 per cent over the past 15 years (Parkin, 2001).

In the UK, cancer of the prostate is fast becoming a major and significant healthcare problem. The NHS will be spending in excess of £55 million per annum to treat men with prostate cancer (Cancer Research UK, 2002). Altogether, one in six (17 per cent) new cases of male cancers in the UK was prostate cancer.

Table 6.6 Prostate cancer: estimates of the numbers of cases and deaths per annum in the USA, UK, EU and the world

Geographical area	Number of cases (per year)	Number of deaths (per year)
USA	198 100 (2001)	31 500 (2001)
UK	21 748 (1997)	9490 (1999)
EU	134 870 (1996)	55 700 (1996)
World	543 000 (2000)	204 000 (2000)

Cancer Research UK (2002).

Histology

Most cases of prostate cancer are adenocarcinomas, and in general they occur in the peripheral zone of the prostate gland. This contrasts with BPH which commonly arises in the central zone of the gland. These neoplastic changes affect the epithelial lining of the prostatic acini; Bostwick and Brewer (1987) have identified premalignant transformation of these cells and have termed it 'prostactic intraepithelial neoplasia' (PIN). Other types of tumour do occur, including small cell and transitional cell cancers, melanoma and sarcoma (Downey, 2000a). Horwich et al. (1995) state that, in 10 per cent of patients who present with signs and symptoms of BPH, there is an incidental finding of prostate cancer in the tissue removed during TURP. Instances of cancer are also detected *post mortem* (Coleman et al., 1993).

Age

Generally speaking, prostate cancer is a disease of older men. In men under 50 years, it is rare; however, more younger middle-aged men are being diagnosed. When men reach the age of 80 years, about 50 per cent have a focus of cancer in their prostate, although only 1 in 25 men will die of the disease (Department of Health, 2000c). Few cases of prostate cancer are registered in men aged under 50 years (Figure 6.1).

Over 50 per cent of cases are registered in men aged 75 years or over; however, this rises to over 95 per cent of men aged over 60 years. As age increases, so too do incidence rates; the higher rates are seen in the older age groups. It is estimated that about a third of men aged 50 years and over will have a small focus of prostatic cancer; this increases to a half when men reach 80 years. Men are therefore more likely to die with prostate cancer rather than from it.

Trends

There are certain trends associated with prostate cancer. There has been a consistent rise in rates in the 1980s, with an increase in the trend in the early

Figure 6.1 Number of new cases and registration rates for prostate cancer by age in the UK. (Source: Cancer Research UK, 2002.)

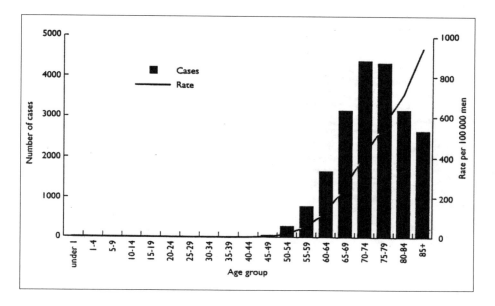

1990s and a decrease in the later 1990s. There may be several reasons for these increases; some may result from a real increase in risk although two other factors also need consideration: an increase in the number of TURPs being performed in the 1980s and the introduction of PSA testing in the 1990s. It could be said that these two factors have contributed to the detection rate of the disease (Cancer Research UK, 2002).

Geographical variation

The highest incidence rates are seen in the USA where world age-standardized rates are in excess of 100 per 10 000 population; this is double the number for reported rates in the UK (Cancer Research UK, 2002). Figure 6.2 demonstrates incidence rates and mortality from a global perspective.

Data from the USA demonstrate that black American men have higher incidence rates than white ones. In addition, the tumours that these men develop are more aggressive and tend to occur at a younger age than in their male counterparts (Kirby and Kirby, 1999). Reported age-standardized incidence rates among black American men are 180 per 10 000 population compared with 105 per 10 000 population among white American men. The lowest rates reported, with fewer than 10 per 10 000 population, are in Far Eastern and Asian countries, e.g. China, Japan and India.

Figure 6.2 World age-standardized incidence rates and mortality rates for prostate cancer in selected countries (estimates are for the year 2000). (Source: Cancer Research UK, 2002.)

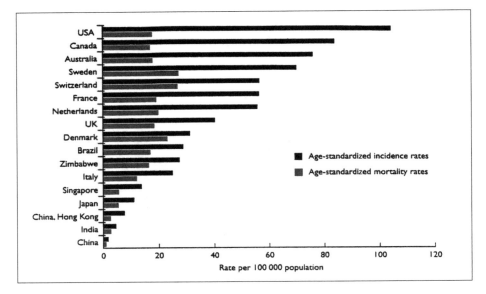

Deprivation

Quinn et al. (2001) and the Scottish Cancer Intelligence Unit (2000) report that, in England, Wales and Scotland, there are higher rates of prostatic cancer in those areas with increased deprivation. However, with regard to mortality rates, the incidence is not associated with deprivation. It is not known to what degree the incidence and survival differences reflect accurate variation in risk by socially deprived group, or any differences that there may be in accessing screening services and/or patient presentation (Cancer Research UK, 2002).

Risk factors

Currently there are few epidemiological data on what preventive strategy can be formed after highlighting the possible risk factors. The data available do not suggest that the possible risk factors substantially influence prostate cancer risk. However, one of the most important risk factors is age: low risk in men under 50 years and increasing risk as the man ages beyond that.

Genetic factors appear to be a predisposing factor with a higher incidence reported in men who have relatives with prostate cancer. What is more significant is that, when a patient has an affected father, brother, grandfather or uncle, there is an eightfold increased risk. In these family groups, the disease develops at an earlier age, and the tumour is more aggressive, which may suggest that a genetic component is influencing the biological actions of the tumour.

Generally speaking, men who live in urban areas have higher mortality rates associated with prostate cancer. In these urban areas, men are exposed to higher levels of environmental pollution, e.g. car fumes, cadmium, chemical carcinogens and possibly chemical fertilizers through food (Fillingham and Douglas, 1997a). Table 6.7 gives some of the possible factors that may increase the risk of prostate cancer.

Table 6.7 Possible factors that may increase the risk of prostate cancer

Factor	Variable
Demographic	• Increasing age • Place of residence
Genetic	• Family history of prostate cancer • Family history of breast cancer • Race – black
Dietary	• High animal fat consumption • Low selenium intake
Occupational	• Cadmium exposure • Radiation exposure • Farming

Source: Cancer Research UK (2002).

As there are variations in incidence around the world, and within countries, and in racial differences, this could imply that risk is affected by ethnicity. However, according to Cancer Research UK (2002), some migrant studies would suggest that environmental factors also have a part to play in increasing the risk of developing prostate cancer, as the rates for migrants from low-risk to high-risk countries increases.

Western diet appears to be a factor that should be considered, because much of the Western diet in developed countries is high in animal fat. Japanese migrants to the USA increase their risk of developing prostate cancer, which could be associated with a change in diet. The high-fat diet consumed in the West may affect the hormone testosterone, which, as has been demonstrated earlier, influences growth and function of the prostate gland. Blumenfeld et al. (2000) suggest that a diet high in vegetables could have a protective effect against the development of prostate cancer.

Symptoms

The symptoms for localized prostate cancer can be the same as for BPH (see earlier discussion of BPH in this chapter). Often, however, localized prostatic cancer is asymptomatic; men with advanced prostate cancer tend to present with back pain which is often associated with skeletal metastases. Downey (2000a) states that approximately 10–15 per cent of men present with symptoms associated with skeletal metastases. However, men with carcinoma of the prostate may have a relatively shorter history of symptoms, e.g. months as opposed to years, which may be the case with BPH.

Staging and grading

The TNM system is used to grade tumours. The system describes the anatomical degree of the disease by using three components:

- T for the primary tumour
- N for the regional lymph nodes
- M for distant metastases

Each of the categories is assigned a number that is related to the extent of disease; this varies depending on the anatomical site and the particular type of malignancy:

- Tis   Carcinoma *in situ*
- T0   No evidence of primary
- Tx   Primary cannot be assessed
- Nx   Nodes cannot be assessed
- Mx   Metastases cannot be assessed
- G1   Well differentiated
- G2   Moderately differentiated
- G3   Poorly differentiated
- G4   Undifferentiated
- pT/N/M   Pathological staging.

The system is a comprehensive one that covers all types and stages of cancer. According to Neal and Hoskin (1997), the TNM system is accepted and recognized by eminent research groups such as the World Health Organization (WHO) and the International Union Against Cancer (UICC).

If the tumour is confined within the prostatic capsule, it is known as 'early disease'. If, however, the disease has spread beyond the prostate gland

and into the surrounding tissue, and there are no other signs that it has spread to other parts of the body, this is known as T3/T4 and can be described as 'locally advanced' disease. Tumours are also graded according to cell structure. The cells are graded from well differentiated, which are the least aggressive, to undifferentiated as in the most aggressive cells.

Screening and diagnosis

Three particular screening tests are used to detect prostate cancer:

- Digital rectal examination (DRE)
- Measurement of PSA
- Transrectal ultrasonography (TRUS).

As most prostate tumours (> 70 per cent: Kirby and Kirby, 1999) develop in the peripheral zone of the gland, many nodules are palpable on DRE. However, if the tumour is palpable, invasion of the prostatic capsule has usually occurred and, if this is the case, more often than not, the tumour is incurable by surgical means. Prostate malignancy is often associated with elevated levels of PSA; in a healthy man the normal value of PSA is 0–4 µg/l. However, there are some drawbacks associated with PSA screening. The results of the test are unreliable if the man has undergone a DRE, has had a urinary catheter passed or has ejaculated before the blood test is taken. TRUS is regarded as a complementary examination to TURP. With all three screening techniques, there are advantages and disadvantages (Table 6.8).

Nurses need to be aware of the advantages and disadvantages of screening for prostate cancer, which is vital if they are to act as the patient's advocate and help him to make the right decision about his health. As a result of the uncertainties surrounding prostate cancer screening, Cancer Research UK (2002) recommend that screening of asymptomatic men should not be undertaken. However, men have a right to request screening and this should be respected, although those men who wish to be screened should be told about the possible consequences of the various screening techniques.

Diagnosis is confirmed by histological evidence. Biopsy of the prostate gland is taken under the guidance of TRUS. Computed tomography or magnetic resonance imaging can confirm staging of the tumour. The degree of PSA elevation also provides information about local tumour stage. A bone scan may be required if there is evidence of metastases; likewise, if metastases are suspected in the lung, a chest radiograph is needed.

Table 6.8 Advantages and disadvantages of the three screening tests

Test	Advantages	Disadvantages
• Prostate-specific antigen (PSA)	• Superior to DRE and TRUS: claimed to be more objective and cost-effective • Some studies have demonstrated that PSA analysis is able to detect prostate cancer better than DRE and, as most of these cancers are localized, they are potentially more curable (Tibblin et al., 1995) • More culturally accepted than DRE	• An elevated serum concentration of PSA is not specific for prostate cancer • Benign prostatic hyperplasia, acute prostatitis and prostatic ischaemia can all cause an elevation of PSA • PSA alone may not always identify men with organ-confined prostatic cancer • PSA alone lacks specificity and sensitivity for an early diagnosis of prostate cancer
• Digital rectal examination (DRE)	• Relatively simple and fast	• Lacks sensitivity for early detection of prostate cancer • May be culturally unacceptable
• Transrectal ultrasonography (TRUS)	• May be more sensitive than DRE • Relatively simple and fast • May be more culturally acceptable than DRE	• Low positive predictive value • Relatively expensive

Treatment

Early disease

There is, at present, no agreement about the treatment for early prostate cancer. However, there are two curative options and men need to consider the following: radical prostatectomy or radical radiotherapy. Treatment options for localized prostate cancer are highlighted in Table 6.9.

The 10-year survival rate for all three options is high (Donovan et al., 1999):

- 'Watchful waiting': 70–90 per cent survival
- Radical prostatectomy: 80–90 per cent
- Radical radiotherapy: 65–90 per cent.

Table 6.9 Treatment options for localized prostate cancer

Watchful waiting	Radical prostatectomy	Radical radiotherapy
• Surveillance • Non-invasive • Metastatic cancer may develop • Uncertainty unacceptable	• Aim to cure • Impotence – up to 80% • Incontinence – up to 20% • Mortality ranges between 0.2 and 1.2%	• Aim to cure • Impotence up to 80% • Incontinence – up to 5% • Long term diarrhoea/bowel problems in up to 10%

Cancer Research UK (2002).

Both curative options have substantial side effects; 'watchful waiting' does not. However, some men may experience significant anxiety and a small proportion may also develop incurable metastatic disease. The nurse must give the patient as much information as possible so that he can take part fully, with full knowledge, in the decision-making process.

Radical prostatectomy

Radical prostatectomy is described as removal of the whole prostate gland, including the capsule (if the cancer remains within the capsule, a TURP is performed). The approach taken for radical prostatectomy is a retropubic approach – the urethral aspects of the prostate are then anastomosed. Often pelvic lymphadenectomy is performed at the same time. The aim is for complete removal of the entire tumour.

Specific preoperative nursing care
A great deal of psychological care is needed for the patient and his family. The fact that the man has cancer is distressing; furthermore, some of the potential complications (e.g. retrograde ejaculation, incontinence) may be a very real concern for him and his partner. The nurse must ensure that the patient and his family are given time to vent any fears or anxieties that they may have; this is also an ideal time for the nurse to correct any misunderstandings. The nurse must explain things to the patient in a language that he understands and the information must be given at a pace that he can manage. To reinforce the point that the nurse is trying to make, the giving of information can be supplemented by written materials.

Bowel preparation must be carried out according to local policy because, during the procedure, the bowel may need to be mobilized. It is important that the nurse ensures that the patient does not become dehydrated during bowel preparation. At all times, the man's dignity must be ensured.

Specific postoperative nursing care

The aim of postoperative nursing care is to promote comfort, relieve anxiety, facilitate urinary output, promote wound healing, monitor and maintain fluid balance, and prevent postoperative complications (e.g. deep vein thrombosis and chest infection). The nurse caring for the patient must therefore be a knowledgeable and skilled practitioner. On return to the ward, the patient will have two urinary catheters *in situ* – a urethral catheter and a urinary catheter – an intravenous drip and two wound drains. The patient may also have central venous access and epidural or patient-controlled analgesia. Pain control is vital and should be assessed as appropriate; monitoring of vital signs is also essential. The nurse must ensure that fluid balance is maintained and bladder irrigation is needed. Hourly urine measurements are made and, if the urine output falls below 30 ml/h, this must be reported to the doctor because this could indicate renal malfunction (Fillingham and Douglas, 1997a).

Fluids should start as soon as bowel sounds have been heard and the patient is able to tolerate them. A light diet can be given after fluids are taken and tolerated, which is often 2–4 days after surgery. The wound drains are cared for and managed according to local policy, i.e. monitoring and recording output, and preventing infection etc. on their removal.

The suprapubic catheter is left in for up to three days and the urethral catheter for up to three weeks. The catheter acts as a splint for the prostatic urethral anastomosis. Prescribed antibiotic therapy is needed, initially intravenously, and then orally to complete the course. After one week (depending on progress), the patient is discharged home and needs information on how to manage the catheter there. Referral to primary nursing services is also needed, i.e. to a district nurse. The patient is readmitted to have the catheter removed – a urethrogram may be needed before its removal (Downey et al., 1997). Unfortunately the patient may have urinary incontinence, so the nurse needs to refer the patient to a continence adviser before, and after, discharge.

Radical radiotherapy

Radiotherapy can be delivered externally or implanted, i.e. the insertion of radioactive pellets of palladium or iodine under ultrasonic control (Blasko et al., 1995). Externally delivered radiotherapy is an ideal treatment option for some patients who are frail, because it does not require hospitalization and there are lower risks of erectile dysfunction. However, Kirby and Kirby (1999) state that it may not eradicate all cancer in every patient and it does it not suppress PSA levels as effectively as surgical intervention. In attempting to downsize the tumour, radiotherapy combined with androgen ablation therapy (bilateral subcapsular orchidectomy) is the treatment of choice.

Implantation of radioactive palladium or iodine is known as brachyther-apy. This technique is relatively new and its effectiveness needs to be analysed using randomized studies comparing brachytherapy with the standard forms of treatment.

There are no studies that have compared radical surgery with radical radiotherapy or 'watchful waiting'. As a result of the absence of empirical data, the treatment options must be fully discussed with the patient, so that he is able to make an informed decision about the proposed management of his illness.

Effects of treatment on the man's sexual health

Prostatic disease can have an effect on a variety of the activities of daily liv-ing; in particular, it can have a profound effect on sexuality. Some people (nurses included) may think that, as prostatic disease affects predominantly older men, they will have few, if any, concerns about their sexuality; such a belief is a myth. It has been discussed earlier that sexuality concerns more than just the sexual act; it concerns and embraces the well-being of the whole person.

Psychological issues must be dealt with and the nurse may feel that he or she is not the appropriate person to address such issues. If this is the case then he or she needs to know who is the most appropriate person for refer-ral, e.g. psychosexual therapist.

Surgical intervention has the potential to affect the man in many ways. Where bilateral subcapsular orchidectomy has been performed, the patient may feel that his body image has been altered. Orchidectomy affects the man's self-image and there are many myths surrounding it, e.g. some men believe (falsely) that removal of the testes will result in a high-pitched voice. The nurse can and must allay the patient's fears and misconceptions. Erectile dysfunction is not a definite complication of bilateral subcapsular orchidec-tomy, but it can happen. The role played by the nurse in explaining about erectile dysfunction has been discussed in detail earlier. After orchidectomy, there is a rise in serum luteinizing hormone-releasing hormone and luteiniz-ing hormone levels; elevation of the latter can result in men experiencing hot flushes and loss of libido. This loss is as much psychological as it is physio-logical. Diminution in sexual desire is frequently associated with depression, which may be how the patient feels if he has prostatic disease. When libido is lowered, several things happen. The patient and partner become aware of a loss of their usual sexual drive. The nurse can encourage the partner of the man to be aware of why his libido may be low. Sensitivity to such things can help couples to understand the difficult time through which they are going.

Many patients (and their partners) benefit from the intervention of a psy-chosexual therapist. The therapist may instigate a cognitive–behavioural and psychodynamic approach to address the problem, with or without the patient's partner.

Retrograde ejaculation can be very distressing physically and psychologically for both the patient and his partner; its impact is even more damaging when the patient has not been told that this is a possibility after surgery. Men who lose the ability to have anterograde ejaculation can retain erectile function and still experience orgasm. When a man does not sense fluid passing through the urethra on ejaculation, he can become alarmed if he has not been warned. A result of this may be that he becomes depressed over the inability to complete this aspect of the male sexual response cycle, and impotence may follow. Retrograde ejaculation is clearly an issue that will concern men who wish to father children. Spark (2000) states that it is possible to retrieve semen that has been ejaculated backward and into the bladder, and use it for insemination. However, the procedure is arduous and time-consuming with little success.

Pelvic radiation rarely results in a reduced sex drive; it may, however, cause the penis to become dry. If this is the case, the patient should be encouraged to use a water-based lubricating gel to aid dryness for both the patient and his partner. Radiotherapy may result in diarrhoea and, as such, could interfere with sexual activity; anti-diarrhoeal medication may be indicated in this case. Treatment to the prostate gland can result in the rectum becoming irritated by the radiotherapy – proctitis; the patient should avoid constipation by taking a high-fibre diet. Thrusting during intercourse can also be painful so a gentler approach to coitus is advocated. Anal intercourse should cease until signs of proctitis have abated and when intercourse resumes it should be gentle.

Stanway (1995) gives practice advice about ways in which some of the difficulties experienced by men with cancer and their partners can be reduced to help overcome them. He clearly states that there is no single answer that will suit everyone, but that patients should at least try some of these approaches:

- Improve communication about sex between yourself and your partner
- Try to give/receive sensual massage
- Learn more about sex; read a good sex manual
- Use more fantasy
- Encourage your partner to contribute more in bed
- Get your partner to learn to stimulate you in the way you like
- Try sex toys
- Try role-playing; act out fantasies.

Health promotion

Screening women for breast cancer has been a very important health activity. Screening men for prostate cancer requires a very different approach. The key question has to be how effective is prostate cancer screening, i.e. PSA measurement? Do the benefits outweigh the potential risks? Sound evidence of benefit must be produced before population screening can be considered. Currently, there is no Government policy on screening because clear benefit has yet to be seen. The benefits of population screening for breast cancer are clearly defined, whereas those for prostate cancer are not (Department of Health, 2000c).

As there is little evidence to suggest that screening for prostate cancer is effective, the main form of prevention is health education/promotion. Any activity undertaken for prostate cancer must highlight the risks and raise awareness about the key symptoms, so that men will be encouraged to visit their GP at an early stage when most prostate cancers can be cured. Nurses in primary care settings, according to Edwards et al. (1999), have a pivotal role to play in health promotion:

- Encourage men to seek advice early for urinary symptoms such as nocturia, difficulty in starting to pass urine, a poor stream or haematuria.
- Identify bladder outflow obstruction through sensitive questioning during routine consultations.
- Refer to appropriate healthcare agency.
- Explain the proposed investigations and interpret the results.
- Explain the proposed treatment options.
- Act as resource, i.e. giving information.

Nurses wishing to provide information for patients should consider the following: patient information should be available in all healthcare settings. The information should cover the basic biology of the prostate gland and its associated organs; the common treatment options and their advantages and disadvantages should also be discussed. Alternative sources of information-giving should also be considered, e.g. Internet access to sites such as CancerHelp UK. Material must be available in languages appropriate to local ethnic minorities. Nurses should also be aware that other sources are available via organizations such as Cancer Research UK, Cancerlink, CancerBACUP and Macmillan Cancer Relief.

Most men die with prostate cancer rather from it. Early detection and treatment of prostatic disease means that more men will have an increase in the quality and quantity of life. Raising this subject can only help men come forward to seek help and advice at an early stage.

Conclusion

Prostatic disease affects the man (and his partner) in many ways. The outcome of treatment can have an overwhelming effect on the quality of life and indeed affects all activities of daily living. The outcome of prostatic disease has specific implications for the quality of the man's sexuality and his sexual health. The nurse, by acting as advocate and encouraging men to seek help and advice at an early stage via innovative and creative approaches to health promotion, can reduce the effects of prostatic disease on a man's sense of well-being.

Although prostatic disease tends to affect elderly men, nurses and other members of the healthcare team must remember that sexual identity, sexual need and the desire for intimacy can continue throughout life. Often, older people are discouraged from seeking help and advice from knowledgeable nurses because of ageist myths, societal stereotypes and the attitudes of those around them.

Nurses have a central role to play in helping older people to express themselves in the way that they choose; this is even more important when the patient is ill. Nurses can help individuals to speak about problems and to deal with them. Nurses should ensure that they feel comfortable speaking about sexuality, that they are open and honest, and give opportunities for patients to talk about sex, and that they construct an atmosphere conducive to discussing personal intimate issues.

Future considerations

Prostatic disease has often been termed a Cinderella disease; however, the future has a more optimistic feel to it. Recently, the UK Department of Health launched a prostate cancer programme for the NHS (Department of Health, 2000c). The document outlines plans for £4.2 million of directly commissioned research, increased by 20-fold compared with 1999/2000. A prostate cancer risk management programme is to be introduced in order to ensure that any man considering a PSA test will be given detailed information to enable him to make an informed choice about whether or not to go ahead with the test. Guidelines are to be produced for GPs about PSA testing and standardized information for patients made available. For those men who wish to have a PSA test, this is now available. The programme has committed the Government to increase the number of urologists by 18 per cent by 2005.

There are no known primary prevention measures that men can take to minimize the risk of developing prostate cancer. However, there is a great deal of ongoing research in order to determine, for example, the effects of diet and how exercise may affect risk (Cancer Research UK, 2000).

Nurses in all healthcare settings can help men to seek advice and support if they are experiencing any prostatic problems. Innovative and creative approaches to raising the issue of prostatic disease can be taken. The nurse must be knowledgeable and confident when discussing this sensitive subject.

CHAPTER SEVEN

Sexually transmitted infections

There has been an unprecedented shift over the past 30 years in the UK in attitudes towards sex and sexuality; the reasons for this are complex and wide ranging. In the UK, sexually transmitted infections (STIs) are common sources of infectious disease. Morbidity and recent Government initiatives have prioritized sexual health as an area for health improvement. There are many STIs that could be addressed in this chapter. HIV is not addressed in detail because it is felt that to discuss HIV and STIs in one chapter would not do justice to either. Only three STIs are discussed:

• Gonorrhoea
• Chlamydial infection
• Syphilis.

Sexually transmitted infections (they used to be referred to as sexually transmitted diseases or STDs) are transmitted through sexual intimacy. For HIV and AIDS there are many other publications that the reader can be directed to concerning these issues (see for example, Adler, 2001; Pratt, 2001; Gazzard, 2002).

It is timely that, with the publication of this text, the British Government has published its first national strategy for sexual health (Department of Health, 2001). In this publication, it states that we have the lowest rate of HIV in western Europe because of various sexual health initiatives, e.g. needle exchange schemes, informing people about risk and open access to genito-urinary medicine (GUM) clinics.

However, regardless of these excellent achievements, there can be no room for complacency. There has been a rise in the number of STIs and unintended pregnancies over the years, and the male population needs to be aware of this. Nurses can ensure that this happens by providing men with the information that they need to protect their health and the health of their partner.

As with various issues dealt with in this text, there is a clear interrelationship of sexual health, poverty and social exclusion. Although the provision of sexual health services remains varied across the UK, a unified and equitable approach should be decided on.

The National Strategy for Sexual Health aims to apply the values and principles of *The NHS Plan* (Department of Health, 2000a) to sexual health in order to redesign services around people who access them. The strategy is ambitious. Other key aims of the strategy are to:

- improve services, information and assistance for all those who need them
- reduce inequalities in sexual health
- enhance health generally, sexual health specifically, and well-being,

The Men's Health Forum (2001) states that although they welcome the National Strategy they would like to see the sexual healthcare needs of men addressed from a gender perspective. They argue that a variety of approaches are needed to ensure that the plan is executed in full for the population as a whole. The needs of men are not the same as those for women, so a gender perspective is necessary. The document defines sexual health as:

> . . . an important part of physical and mental health. It is a key part of our identity as human beings together with the fundamental human rights to privacy, a family life and living free from discrimination. Essential elements of good sexual health are equitable to relationships and sexual fulfilment with access to information and services to avoid the risks of unintended pregnancy, illness or disease.

This all-embracing definition of sexual health makes a statement about the wide range of sexual health components, which must be praised, because often definitions of sexual health fail to do this. However, the rest of the document appears to disregard this remarkable definition, and concentrates on prevention and treatment of STIs and HIV. The strategy should have taken the opportunity of including initiatives that advance positive sexual health, as opposed to focusing on what takes place when things go wrong for people. More emphasis is needed on issues such as sexual dysfunction and sex education.

Nevertheless, the strategy recognizes that sexual health and HIV services are in need of modernization, and that there has been a rising prevalence of STIs and HIV. Plans are made in the document to address these issues.

Poor sexual health can have serious consequences for individuals and societies. The result of an unintended pregnancy or STI can have a long-lasting effect on a person's life. Evidence suggests that there has been an increase, over the past decade, in the number of visits paid to GUM clinics; this number has almost doubled and stands at over 1 million per annum (Department of Health, 2001). However, the increase in the number of visits may be the result of several factors, e.g. people may feel more at ease to consult nurses and other healthcare professionals at GUM clinics because of their concerted efforts to reduce the stigma associated with attending these clinics.

It is relatively much easier to encourage men to attend a GUM clinic than to consult their GP if they have any genitourinary symptoms such as urethral discharge or dysuria. The GUM clinic is able to make an on-the-spot diagnosis from microscopic examination of secretions obtained from urethral swabs (Curtis et al., 1996). A GUM clinic, with the man's consent, will often routinely test for a wide range of STIs.

Between 1995 and 2000, the new episodes of STIs seen at GUM clinics in England, Wales and Northern Ireland rose from 887 760 to 1 185 285 (Public Health Laboratory Service or PHLS, 2001):

- Uncomplicated gonorrhoea rose by 102 per cent (29 per cent since 1999)
- Chlamydial infection increased by 107 per cent (18 per cent since 1999)
- Syphilitic infections increased up 145 per cent (57 per cent since 1999).

There can be many reasons why there has been an increase in the numbers of people being seen in GUM clinics and diagnosed with an STI:

- An increase in transmission of STIs
- Improved acceptability of GUM clinic services
- Greater public awareness of some STIs
- Greater health professional awareness of some STIs
- Developments in diagnostic test sensitivity.

The data collected from GUM clinics underestimate the number of cases of STIs in the population as a whole. This is because the diagnosis of an STI in a non-GUM setting is not recorded in the GUM clinic data set unless the patient is referred to the GUM clinic by a healthcare professional. Furthermore, the accessibility and uptake of GUM services may influence the number of diagnoses made, i.e. access to GUM clinics may be difficult in some areas where public transport is poor or when opening times are restrictive. Finally, some infections such as chlamydial infection and gonorrhoea may be asymptomatic and therefore not diagnosed.

Brief history of sexually transmitted infections

STIs have a long history; they are mentioned in the Bible and there is evidence of them being referenced in ancient Chinese and Greek medical texts. Myth and superstition often influenced the early treatment of STIs. Some typical preventive procedures in the early years included the wrapping of sex organs in wool, cold baths and abstinence from sexual intercourse (Evans, 1994). Walking barefoot on a cold floor or the placing of leeches on the scrotum was the treatment for gonorrhoea. For many years, according to Gelbart (1999), the treatment options for syphilis were mercurially based; in the 1800s arsenic-based preparations were the drug of choice.

Many hospitals refused to accept patients with venereal diseases; however, some time after the fifteenth century, specialist hospitals were set up to care for patients with these diseases. In Britain these hospitals were known as lock hospitals.

Often GUM clinics are still tucked away in hospital basements or towards the rear of the hospital's main entrance, which may give the impression that genitourinary medicine is a 'Cinderella' service (Jones M, 1994). Labels such as venereal diseases (VD), sexually transmitted diseases (STDs) and 'special clinics' only added to the stigma surrounding genitourinary medicine. A concerted effort has been made over the past 20 years or so to move away from such labels and to a broader focus surrounding sexual health.

In the 1400s a pandemic erupted in the form of a new deadly disease – syphilis. Millions of Europeans were affected by *Treponema pallidum* – the causative organism of syphilis. Syphilis, one of the earliest STIs to be discovered, was known by 400 different names. Blame theory appears to be a reason why so many names associated with syphilis are country names, 'Polish illness', 'German pox', 'French pox' and the 'Portuguese disease' – probably as a result of transmission by soldiers from one country to another.

During the First World War there was an increase in the number of STIs and this increase forced the government of the day to take decisive action to limit the disease. They did this in the form of legislation. The Public Health (Venereal Diseases) Regulations of 1916 were introduced. The regulations ensured that the public would be entitled to free and confidential treatment of STIs; attendance was voluntary. The Second World War brought with it a large increase in the number of STIs, not only in the UK but worldwide. Penicillin was discovered and was extensively used to treat the many soldiers who had contracted syphilis.

Although the discovery of penicillin in medicine was generally welcomed, it is possible that its arrival, combined with the free and confidential service offered to patients, may also have led to an expansion in sexual freedom. The 1960s saw the arrival of the contraceptive pill, which resulted in a reduction in the use of barrier methods of contraception such as condoms; the outcome of this was an increase in the numbers of STIs contracted.

What was also significant during this period was that the number of cases of gonorrhoea reflected the increase in the number of casual sexual encounters people were having. Furthermore, a more sinister occurrence emerged – there was a new wave of STIs, e.g. chlamydial infection, non-specific urethritis, genital warts and genital herpes. Garrett (1994) reports that, from the 1970s, there was a steep rise in the numbers of gay men with STIs compared with the population as a whole.

The 1980s saw the arrival of HIV and, for the first time in decades, the human race was, and still is, faced by a disease that is pandemic in nature. HIV infection is loaded with myth and stigma and is potentially life threatening.

healthcare initiatives that aim to limit and reduce the spread of STIs are important, not only to combat diseases such as gonorrhoea and syphilis, but also to reduce the number of cases of HIV because STIs also allow the transmission of the virus. healthcare professionals must be prepared to discuss sexuality openly with their patients if they are to encourage them to modify their sexual behaviour and reduce the stigma associated with HIV (Gelbart, 1999).

Nursing care of the patient with an STI

The nursing care of any patient with an STI requires the nurse to be sensitive to the patient's condition. Patients are often embarrassed and very anxious and there is much that the nurse can do to alleviate this. Patients may be feeling guilty (Walsh, 1997) and marital difficulties may arise if one partner infects the other. There is a social stigma attached to STIs, so confidentiality must be maintained at all times. The nurse must adhere to the guiding principles laid down by the Nursing and Midwifery Council (NMC, 2002). Each patient presents with individual needs and a thorough nursing assessment is necessary, be this in a hospital setting, a GUM clinic or an outpatient setting.

The nurse must take a detailed sexual health history. It is crucial that this is conducted in such a way as to elicit as much information as possible. It should be explained clearly to the patient why the sexual health history is needed. The nurse needs to make a diagnosis in order to confirm the presence of an STI. In some centres this may be the sole responsibility of the nurse, with referral to medical staff or other appropriate agencies as necessary.

A physical examination has to be done to ascertain the extent of the disease. The nurse must promote comfort for the patient, educate the patient and prevent infection to other individuals (Roper et al., 1996). All nurses should practise universal precautions for all patients. There is no need for extra precautions such as isolation when caring for patients with an STI in a general ward setting; the nurse must provide good-quality care to all patients.

When promoting comfort, the physical and psychological aspects of care must be considered. Physical aspects include comforting measures such as the administration of analgesia, the correct positioning of limbs, and support of the limbs if the patient has arthralgia, specifically related to STIs such as syphilis. The major goals are the relief of pain or discomfort, symptom control, control of infection and prevention of transmission (Scherer and Timby, 1995).

Full explanations of diagnostic tests, e.g. blood tests, possibly lumbar puncture, and radiological investigations, may be needed. In patients with syphilis, lumbar puncture can help the practitioner to rule out other causes of nervous system dysfunction, and is indicated in cases of neurosyphilis to confirm the diagnosis or exclude asymptomatic neurosyphilis (Wisdom, 1992). Explanation enables the nurse to gain informed consent from the patient and helps to allay fears and anxieties. Good communication skills are needed to ensure effective two-way exchange of information (Sutherland, 1996). While conducting the physical examination, the practitioner should strive to maintain the patient's dignity and privacy.

Contact tracing

Contact tracing is needed in order to treat contacts (if necessary) and prevent the disease from spreading. Usually, one individual has sole responsibility for this task. The nurse, however, may be instrumental in gaining vital information about the sexual practices of patients and their partners. Interviewing patients about their contacts requires effective communication skills, tact and sensitivity. It is important to get in touch with the patient's sexual contacts and advise them to attend a clinic as soon as possible, in order to reduce the number of subsequent infections. The aim is to regulate the disease within the community, as well as to care for the health of individuals who are symptomless and who may be unaware that they have an infection. The reason for contact tracing must be explained to the patient and his partner if co-operation is to occur.

Prevention and education go hand in hand. The nurse must apply scrupulous infection control practices in order to prevent cross-infection. She or he must adhere to policy and procedure. The nurse will be called on to give information and advice at various levels. Safer sex practices have to be addressed if the risk of transmission is to be reduced.

Once the patient has commenced drug therapy, he must be encouraged to complete the course of antibiotics. The patient needs to be informed of the reasons why he requires antibiotic therapy and of the potential side effects of such drugs. Sexual intercourse must be avoided until the patient is told that the disease has been successfully treated. Again, the skills of the nurse and the way they are used could have a positive or negative effect on the outcome.

Tracing and notifying sexual partners is a vital aspect of any STI control programme. Individuals must be encouraged to inform their partner(s) of their condition. In most GUM clinics, the health adviser adopts the role of contact tracer. Contact tracers need to be tactful and sensitive, and to have excellent communication skills. The reason why contact tracing is required needs to be explained fully to the individual because this will encourage co-operation.

Chlamydial infection

Taylor-Robinson (1996) states that chlamydial infection is the most common curable STI in the developed world. It is so common that the Health Education Authority (1992) believe that it is the most widespread of human infections – more prevalent than the common cold. The bacterium responsible for causing chlamydial infection is *Chlamydia trachomatis*; these micro-organisms live as parasites within cells and can infect the genitals; it also has the potential to infect the throat and eye.

The consequences of untreated chlamydial infection can be serious for men and their female partners. If untreated, the infection primarily causes pelvic inflammatory disease (PID). Stamm et al. (1984) estimate that 30 per cent of untreated or inadequately treated women will present with PID. The effects of chlamydial infection can result in infertility and ectopic pregnancy. Rooney and Robinson (1997) state that the main cause of epididymitis in young men is *Chlamydia*.

Epidemiology

The number of cases of chlamydial infection reported by GUM clinics has risen steadily and, since the mid-1990s, there has been an increase – 76 per cent since 1995 (Pimenta and Fenton, 2001). Between 1999 and 2000 there was a 20 per cent rise in chlamydial infections in men. In 20- to 24-year-old men the rates of chlamydial infection are 579 per 100 000 of the male population (Eurosurveillance, 2001). During the year 2000 in England, the rates in both males and females were highest in London – 186 and 214 per 100 000, respectively.

The substantial rise in the numbers of cases notified may, however, be related to the increased availability and uptake of testing. Coupled with this, it may be that diagnostic testing has become more sensitive, but the concurrent rise in the numbers of other STIs may indicate that there has been an increase in the number of people who practise unsafe sex.

Clinical manifestations

Many cases of chlamydial infection remain undetected because up to 70 per cent of women and 50 per cent of men who are infectious may be asymptomatic (Cates and Wasserheit, 1991). It is therefore a serious public health problem.

Individuals with a chlamydial infection present with symptoms that are similar to those of other STIs. Jovanovich (1999) states that chlamydial infection and other STIs often coexist, e.g. with gonorrhoea, and, as such, patients are pre-emptively treated for both infections.

Men may present with any combination of symptoms as summarized below:

- dysuria or frequency of micturition
- penile discharge, which can be clear, thin and milky-white
- burning and itching close to the urethra
- lower abdominal pain and abdominal tenderness
- testicular pain, tenderness and swelling
- an unusual anal discharge.

In 75 per cent of male patients, the primary site for infection is in the urethra. The infection also has the potential to ascend to the prostate gland, epididymis and the testes. Chlamydial infection is also the most common cause of non-specific urethritis (NSU) in the male.

Diagnosis

Making a sound diagnosis depends on systematic investigations. An in-depth accurate history needs to be taken from the patient to elicit important data. Adler (2000) suggests that men who have a high-risk profile (men who are susceptible to contracting chlamydial infection) have the following:

- a change of partner
- multiple sexual partners
- recurrent symptoms
- symptoms in a partner
- general symptoms such as abdominal pain, rash and arthralgia.

A comprehensive physical examination is needed to detect those who may present with a concurrent STI. When examining the male patient, the nurse should examine the penis, and a urethral swab and a urine specimen should be taken. It is best if the patient refrains from micturition for about 4 hours before the sample is taken in order to prevent the washing away of any specimens in the urine. After examining the penis, the nurse should then conduct an examination of the pubic hair, the scrotum, the nearby skin and the perianal area.

There are many tests available to ascertain whether the patient has contracted *Chlamydia*; these tests have improved and continue to improve. It must be noted that there is no single test that has the ability to identify all occurrences of chlamydial infection.

Treatment

The first choice of treatment for chlamydial infection is antibiotic therapy – the tetracyclines, i.e. oxytetracycline or doxycycline (Adler, 2000). For those allergic to the tetracyclines, erythromycin may be prescribed. The antibiotics are often prescribed for a 7-day period.

Screening for *Chlamydia*

There are many debates over a national screening programme to detect chlamydial infection. The aim of screening is to find undiagnosed, asymptomatic cases, and thus stop the long-term sequelae and decrease prevalence of the infection in the population. Although it is noted that screening has the potential to save lives or improve the quality of life through early detection of a serious condition, it is not without shortcomings. With any screening programme there is an irreducible minimum of false positives – incorrectly reported as having the condition – and false negatives – incorrectly reported as not having the condition. According to Herrmann et al. (1991), if screening is to be an appropriate intervention, certain criteria need to be satisfied:

- The condition or its outcomes need to be a serious problem
- There must be a latent or early symptomatic phase
- An effective treatment must be available
- The method of testing must be acceptable to the population.

Screening for chlamydial infection meets most of these criteria. What is unknown is whether testing is acceptable to the population.

Female screening programmes are often seen as attractive to policymakers because women often congregate in health settings that are already functioning, e.g. gynaecology, well woman, antenatal, family planning and termination clinics, as opposed to men, who are often difficult to access. There are problems about how to access men for screening; however, men's health is just as important as women's and curbing an STI is more effective through screening of both sexes.

To this end, the UK has established a national screening programme with an expert advisory group. Some concerns about the implementation of a national screening programme are centred round the issue of antibiotic resistance, if a national screening programme were to be established.

Health education

Patients should be encouraged to tell their partners of the diagnosis and encourage the partners to have a check-up even if they are asymptomatic. Nurses must advise patients not to engage in sexual activity until they have been re-tested and there is no evidence of infection.

Patients should be told that chlamydial infection can be prevented by the use of barrier contraceptives and that the test used for diagnosis and the treatment are simple and effective. It is important that patients are informed of when they need to return for follow-up tests.

In summary, chlamydial infections are very often asymptomatic; a large proportion of the infected population remains undiagnosed, with the consequence that this increases the challenge to primary prevention. Nurses are ideally placed to address these issues with other healthcare professionals and their patients.

Chlamydial infection is a significant threat to public health and, as such, a proactive programme of active case finding and comprehensive partner notification is needed in order to reduce the numbers of people infected. Currently, the detection of chlamydial infection is often limited to specialist services such as GUM clinics. To reduce the number of cases, innovative activities must be undertaken to detect use of other health services by those who are infected, other than the men attending GUM clinics. Screening programmes are still under investigation, e.g. the national screening programme funded by the Department of Health. The outcomes of any investigation need to be given careful consideration by policymakers before there is any commitment to suggestions of a national screening programme.

Syphilis

Syphilis has existed in Europe since the time of Columbus, although the causative organism, *Treponema pallidum*, was not identified until 1905. In 1909 Ehrlich, a German bacteriologist, developed Salvarsan (an organic arsenic or arsphenamine). At the time this was the standard medication for syphilis; however, it was a very toxic treatment. Salvarsan was replaced by neoarsphenamine in 1912. The route of administration was via injection and the course of treatment lasted 12 months. The drug of choice today is procaine penicillin.

Syphilis is relatively uncommon in the UK. Where there are outbreaks of syphilis in England, e.g. in Bristol, this was associated with heterosexually acquired infection, commercial sex work and 'crack' cocaine use; however, cases in Brighton, Manchester and London were among men who have sex with men, some of whom had a concurrent HIV infection (PHLS, 2001).

Epidemiology

Most cases of syphilis among men occur in the most sexually active age group. Epidemiological surveillance lasting over a decade demonstrates that the rates of syphilis in males aged between 20 and 40 years has increased sharply since 1996. In England, between 1998 and 2000, the numbers of men diagnosed with infectious syphilis (primary or secondary) rose by 150 per cent (PHLS, 2001). In the male population, those aged between 25 and 44 years in Northern Ireland, Wales and England accounted for the highest number of men who had syphilis. The highest rates were seen in London with 2.9 per 100 000 people infected and in the north west of the country where 2.0 per 100 000 population were infected with syphilis.

There may be several reasons for the increase in the rate of syphilis:

- More sensitive detection methods
- Increased awareness of syphilis among the general public and healthcare professionals
- Safer sex techniques not being performed
- Health promotion and education programmes failing.

The reason why men feature more than women in the data on syphilitic infection may be that most of the data point to an increase in the number of men who have sex with men. Diagnosis of syphilis declined in the early to mid-1980s, which coincided with an emerging awareness of HIV transmission, adoption of safer sex practices, and a parallel fall in the number of HIV transmissions in men who have sex with men. However, the trend appears to be changing. Men who have sex with men represent the highest rates seen at GUM clinics in London – 2.9 men per 100 000 of the population.

Transmission

Syphilis is caused by the bacterium *Treponema pallidum*, which is classified as a spirochaete. This type of bacterium can infect any organ or tissue in the body, and has the potential to travel to a variety of sites via the bloodstream; for this reason, it has the ability to bring about a wide range of symptoms. Treponemal spirochaetes are slender, spiral organisms with approximately 8–15 coils evenly spaced 1 μm apart, the entire length being 5–15 μm (Morello et al., 1998). They are very slim with multi-layered cell membranes below the cell wall and six flagellum-like fibrils between the cell wall and membrane. Treponemal spirochaetes have a distinctive drifting motility and curve in a graceful manner with slow, undulating movements.

Syphilis is passed on principally during sexual intercourse. The organism is passed from person to person through open lesions on the skin or mucous membranes. Infection takes place at the site of inoculation; a small abrasion or sore is more often than not the site of entry, because the organism cannot break through undamaged mucous membranes. The disease can also be passed to unborn children via the placenta, when it is known as congenital syphilis. A child born with this disease may develop many handicaps and defects.

The incubation period for syphilis ranges from 9 to 90 days (Adler, 2000). The spirochaete pierces damaged mucous membranes and is then able to circulate via the lymphatic system and blood. It needs a moist, dark environment to live and is sensitive to sunlight, antiseptics and air. Hence, it does not live long outside the host; it is a delicate organism requiring particular conditions in which to mature. If untreated the disease progresses through four phases: primary, secondary, latent and tertiary. It may live on for many years and the infected person may be asymptomatic. Throughout the primary and secondary stages, the spirochaete is transmitted exclusively by direct contact.

Screening

Syphilis has such serious effects on the developing foetus that all pregnant women are screened antenatally. Any woman who tests positive to the presence of antibodies for syphilis can be treated during the pregnancy and the foetus can be treated *in utero*. Referral should be made to a GUM clinic for appropriate treatment (Forster et al., 1999).

All patients attending GUM clinics are checked for syphilis serology (Curtis et al., 1996). All blood donors and selected hospital patients (i.e. those who may need neurological or psychiatric assessment) are screened for syphilis (Adler, 2000). This approach to screening for syphilis provides a satisfactory insight into the prevalence of the infection.

Diagnosis

As with all STIs, in order to make a diagnosis, an in-depth patient history is vital. A full physical examination is important and the nurse needs to check, in particular, for skin rashes or any genital ulcers.

There are a number of tests for syphilis. However, *T. pallidum* is not always an easy organism to recognize. Microscopy using dark-ground illumination allows identification of the spirochaete. The Wassermann reaction identifies the presence of *T. pallidum* by means of a complement fixation test. Complement is a component of plasma that enhances antibody function, and is a complex of proteins that facilitates either phagocytosis or puncture of the bacterial cell membrane (Walsh, 1997). Generally, however, this test has been replaced by simpler and less expensive tests.

At the moment, the Wassermann reaction may be used as a preliminary screening test, but a more precise test is needed to confirm the presence of *T. pallidum*. The principal screening tests for syphilis include the VDRL (Venereal Disease Reference Laboratory) and RPR (rapid plasma reagin) tests. These tests are called flocculation tests: the serum is tested to find out whether there has been an antibody–antigen reaction in response to infectious micro-organisms (McCance and Huether, 1998). Although these tests are sensitive to antibodies, they are influenced by the stage of the disease, e.g. in primary syphilis the antibody titre is often low.

Clinical manifestations

Primary syphilis

During the primary stage, a small painless red macule appears, known as a chancre; this develops at the site of infection, and may enlarge and develop through a papular stage. Erosion occurs and it forms a round, indurated, painless ulcer. If left untreated, this ulcer heals spontaneously in about three weeks. The sites of primary syphilis are divided into genital and extragenital and are listed below (Adler, 2000):

- Genital
  - shaft of penis
  - coronal sulcus
  - glans penis
  - prepuce
  - urethral meatus
  - anal margin/canal
  - rectum
- Extragenital
  - lip
  - tongue
  - mouth, throat, tonsil
  - fingers
  - eyelid
  - nipple
  - any part of the skin or mucous membrane.

The chancre, which is highly infectious and has numerous spirochaetes present within it, may cause enlargement of local lymph nodes. At this point, the spirochaetes have already travelled to other parts of the body. The chancre may go unnoticed, depending on the site, because it is painless.

Secondary syphilis

The secondary stage is the dissemination phase. This stage often occurs 1–3 months after the initial infection and the patient may complain of the following:

- Flu-like symptoms
- Anorexia
- Sore throat
- Malaise
- Lymphadenopathy
- Hair loss.

During this stage, the patient develops systemic symptoms, such as a rash. The rash can occur at several sites, e.g. the palms of the hands, the trunk of the body and the soles of the feet, and usually heals, although it may relapse. It is usually non-itchy and symmetrical in appearance. Adler (2000) describes the papular lesions as coppery red and, very rarely, pustular. Further features may also occur and these present as shallow ulcers in the genital mucosa together with formation of condylomata lata – a wart-like growth around the genitalia. Micro-organism activity is very intense at this stage and as such the person is highly infectious.

The sites and types of lesion associated with secondary syphilis are listed in Table 7.1; 75–80 per cent of the clinical features seen in secondary syphilis are skin lesions (Adler, 2000).

Table 7.1 Sites and types of lesion associated with secondary syphilis

Clinical feature	Frequency of occurrence (%)
Skin lesions	75–80
Mucous membrane lesions	30
Generalized lymphadenopathy	50–60
Arthritis, arthralgia Hepatitis Renal disease Ophthalmological involvement Neurological disease	Rare

Latent syphilis

If the disease is untreated, the patient passes into the latent stage. The latent period is often symptom free and can go on for several years. However, serology and blood tests will remain positive for antibodies to *T. pallidum*. Although the patient is asymptomatic he still harbours the infection but at this stage he will no longer be sexually infectious.

Tertiary syphilis

The tertiary stage of syphilis is characterized by a severe and irreversible disease of the nervous system, heart and aorta. Aneurysm of the ascending aorta, aortic regurgitation and coronary ostial stenosis are manifestations of cardiac and aortic disease. The diseases associated with the nervous system manifest themselves as general paralysis of the insane and tabes dorsalis. The blood vessels become damaged and there is a poor blood supply to the tissues. Areas of necrosis known as 'gummas' may occur in several tissues, including the bones. Not all patients progress to the tertiary stage. Below is a guide to the types of syphilis that may result if the disease is left untreated.

- Gummatous syphilis (15 per cent)
- Cardiovascular syphilis (10 per cent)
- Neurosyphilis (10 per cent)
- No clinical sequelae (65 per cent).

Tertiary syphilis, or the third stage, may not always follow the latent stage; in 30 per cent of cases there is spontaneous recovery (Adler, 2000). Factors that determine the effects of syphilis (if the individual has been unable to fight off infection) include:

- The degree of the original infection
- The general health of the person
- The body sites affected.

The body sites affected include the heart, blood vessels, bone, spinal cord and brain. When the brain is involved, a degenerative condition called parenchymatous general paresis of neurosyphilis occurs. The pathological lesion in tertiary syphilis is a chronic granuloma called a gumma. This area of tissue (the gumma) becomes necrotic, resulting in ischaemia. Symptoms include:

- ¥ Intellectual deficits
- Memory loss

- Loss of muscle function
- Loss of speech
- Convulsions
- Ataxia.

As a result of the widespread use of antibiotics in the treatment of syphilis, it is very rare to find patients who have progressed to the tertiary stage. However, in elderly people, as a result of misdiagnosis, there may be a low incidence of tertiary syphilis (Bremmer and Radcliffe, 1993). Weston (1999) recommends that nurses who are caring for elderly people should familiarize themselves with the signs and symptoms of tertiary syphilis in order to prevent misdiagnosis.

Treatment

The typical treatment for syphilis is procaine penicillin. Each trust has its own favoured regimen, but the regimen is also dependent on the stage of the disease. Where patients are allergic to penicillin, erythromycin or tetracycline may be given. Adler (2000) advocates the use of procaine penicillin in primary and secondary syphilis over 10 days, but most institutions now think that the course of treatment should last for 14 days to have full effect. The drug is administered via the intramuscular route.

The nurse has a vital role to play in making certain that the patient appreciates the importance of attending daily for the injection. As the period in which the patient needs to attend includes a weekend, the nurse must arrange for the injection to be given (if he is attending a GUM clinic) by another nurse in another department. Confidentiality must be paramount at all times. During the later stage, when the patient has been diagnosed for less than two years, the same regimen is used. If the individual has been diagnosed for longer than two years, 3.6 g is given for 21 days. When the individual presents with symptoms of neurosyphilis or cardiovascular syphilis, penicillin is still given for 21 days but oral prednisolone is added for one day before and two days after; prednisolone is also indicated where a hypersensitivity reaction, resulting from the presence of spirochaetes, is suspected. Where gummatous syphilis is evident, penicillin is given for 15 days and the prognosis depends on the extent of the lesions (Peate, 1998). Figure 7.1 considers the stages and associated symptoms of syphilis.

The progress of treated syphilis depends on the stage of the disease and the degree of tissue damage. Effective treatment of primary and secondary syphilis and latent asymptomatic neurosyphilis can stop progression of the disease. The inflammatory process is generally halted, but the tissue damage may be too far advanced for any improvement in symptoms.

Primary stage
Chancre
Local lymph nodes
enlargement

Secondary stage
Dissemination
Rash
Generalized lymphadenopathy
General malaise
Pyrexia
Sore throat
Headache
Renal disease
Syphilitic meningitis
Hepatitis
Iridocyclitis
Chorodorentinitis

Latent stage
Asymptomatic

Tertiary stage
Skin lesions
Dysarthia
General paralysis of the insane
Tabes dorsalis
Aortitis

Table 7.1 Stages and symptoms of syphilis.

Jarisch–Herxheimer reaction

Some patients with syphilis may exhibit a systemic reaction to drug therapy – the Jarisch–Herxheimer reaction. If this occurs, the patient may develop fever, excessive sweating and a headache 2–12 hours after commencing treatment, and may need to seek medical advice. The patient should be told to rest, self-administer an antipyretic and increase his fluid input.

Follow-up

The nurse must ensure that the patient understands that he will have to return to the GUM clinic (or the appropriate other department) for follow-up treatment. At each visit he will be clinically examined and have blood tests, i.e. VDRL. It is possible for the patient to relapse. The follow-up is as shown below:

- Monthly for three months
- Three-monthly after three months of treatment
- Two years after the start of treatment.

To summarize, the number of cases of syphilis is increasing for a variety of reasons. As a result of the blanket screening approach in the UK, we are able to monitor the disease. Furthermore, syphilis can easily be treated and, as such, the devastating manifestations of the disease rarely occur.

Each nurse has a crucial role to play in ensuring that the patient with syphilis receives high-quality, effective nursing care. The nurse possesses many skills to ensure that this becomes a reality. Syphilis, if treated at an early stage, has an excellent prognosis. However, if left untreated, damage can occur, both physically and psychologically. Syphilis is primarily transmitted sexually. Caring for patients with syphilis provides the nurse with many opportunities to enhance comfort, prevent infection and educate at all levels.

Gonorrhoea

Gonorrhoea is caused by the bacterium *Neisseria gonorrhoeae* (more commonly referred to as the gonococcus); this infection is universally common and extremely contagious. The infection contaminates mucosal surfaces of the genitourinary tract, rectum, tonsils, conjunctival sac and pharynx, and spreads from tissue to tissue.

The incubation period for gonorrhoea is relatively short, compared with syphilis. Symptoms such as discharge and dysuria can occur in some cases within 24 hours of infection. Gonorrhoea is extremely infectious and, in men, there is a possibility of one in three of contracting the infection from a single sexual encounter with an infected person.

Gonorrhoea is transmitted almost exclusively through sexual contact. In the UK it is one of the most widespread infections (McMillan and Scott, 2000). After many years with a falling incidence, primarily as a result of the onset of HIV in the 1980s, more articulate health education programmes, improved ways of treating the infection and better methods of contact tracing, there now appears to be an increase in the number of cases.

Risk factors include the following:

- Living in an inner city
- Coming from a disadvantaged background
- Being single
- Having had a first sexual encounter at an early age
- Having a history of STIs.

Epidemiology

Incidence rates of gonorrhoea fell after the Second World War largely as a result of the emergence of antibiotics and, as with chlamydial infection, the rates increased during the 1960s.

Between 1999 and 2000 the number of cases of uncomplicated gonorrhoea in males rose from 10 959 to 14 350, which reflects a rise of 31 per cent.
In men who have sex with men, the rates increased from 1861 to 2822 (a rise
of 52 per cent) between 1990 and 2000. This rise was considerably larger
than that seen in men generally. Outbreaks of gonorrhoea occurred in
Manchester, Brighton and London in men who have sex with men (PHLS,
2002). The highest rates of infection occur in young men aged between 20
and 24 years (218 per 100 000 of population)

The continued rise in the diagnoses of STIs over the past six years may
be attributed to the increasing practice of unsafe sexual behaviour,
predominantly in young heterosexuals, and homosexual and bisexual men.
As a result of the longer-term complications related to untreated STIs, as well
as their role in aiding HIV transmission, the data presented here suggest that
nurses must improve current STI prevention strategies if the incidence of
STIs is to fall.

Clinical manifestations

Clinical manifestations of gonorrhoea can be classified as local or systemic,
and uncomplicated or complicated. In males, urethral infection is symptomatic in 90 per cent of cases. The patient with an uncomplicated local
infection presents with a purulent or mucopurulent discharge and/or
dysuria.

The incubation period for males is 3–10 days. If left untreated, urethritis
persists for 3–7 weeks; most men are asymptomatic after three months. Over
50 per cent of men will experience a marked dysuria.

Symptoms of anorectal gonorrhoea can range from a mild anal pruritis,
mucopurulent rectal discharge or slight bleeding, to severe rectal pain, tenes-
mus and constipation. Physical examination with a proctoscope may reveal
anal erythema, discharge and evidence of mucosal damage. Rectal infection
is often asymptomatic.

Gonococcal pharyngitis occurs after performing fellatio on an infected
partner. There may be a pyrexia, lymphadenopathy and tonsillitis. Over half
of the cases of this type of infection are asymptomatic. Symptomatic pharyngitis may be indistinguishable from any other bacterial infection.

The eye is another site that may lead to uncomplicated local infection, in
particular conjunctivitis. According to McCance and Huether (1998), this
type of infection is rare in adults.

Localized gonococcal infection can be complicated by prostatitis, epididymitis, lymphangitis and urethral stricture in males. Individuals who are
infected and untreated are at risk of developing disseminated gonococcal
infection, although this is rare – less than 1 per cent of cases (McMillan and

Scott, 2000). Unilateral epididymo-orchitis is the most common complication; prompt treatment is needed if abscess formation is to be avoided.

Diagnosis

Clinical signs and symptoms are not sufficient for the differential diagnosis of gonococcal infections. Microscopic evaluation of a Gram-stained smear of urethral exudate is needed. When oral or anal infection is suspected, material for culture should be obtained from the pharynx and rectum. McMillan and Scott (2000) suggest that this should be done on two occasions, because infection in these sites is more difficult to obtain. In practice, however, this may be done only once, because the patient may not return to the GUM clinic for a second test.

Treatment

A single dose of antibiotics is the usual treatment for uncomplicated gonorrhoea – ciprofloxacin 250 mg. Often, treatment is also given to cover other coexisting STIs, e.g. chlamydial infection, i.e. doxycycline 200 mg once, then 100 mg once a day for 10 days.

Conclusion

Throughout history, infectious diseases have endangered humans. STIs have been mentioned in the Bible and there is reference to them in ancient Chinese and Greek medical texts. Myth and superstition influenced the early treatment of STIs. The discovery of penicillin in the 1930s resulted in it being used extensively to treat soldiers with syphilis. However, the arrival of penicillin, a free and confidential venereal disease service and the contraceptive pill may have led to an increase in sexual freedom and, therefore, an increase in the numbers of STIs. The 1980s saw new cases of HIV and AIDS and for a time the number of STI cases began to decline; however, they appear to have increased over the last few years as has the number of cases of HIV in the heterosexual population.

This chapter considered three STIs – chlamydial infection, syphilis and gonorrhoea. HIV was not discussed and the reader is urged to consult other texts to learn more about this complex infection.

Chlamydial infection is the most common bacterial STI and is the leading preventable cause of infertility. The causative organism, *Chlamydia trachomatis*, localizes to epithelial tissue and has the ability to spread throughout the urogenital tract. Chlamydial infection is susceptible to inexpensive antibiotic therapy. As a result of the asymptomatic nature of chlamydial infection and the potential sequelae of untreated infections, debate is currently centred on screening the population as a whole.

The number of cases of syphilis in the UK has risen over the past five years. Shortly after infection, syphilis becomes systemic. There are four stages of the disease:

- Primary syphilis (with a chancre at the site of infection)
- Secondary syphilis (systemic spread to all body systems)
- Latent syphilis (minimal symptoms and the development of skin lesions)
- Tertiary syphilis (the most devastating stage – destruction of bone, skin, and soft and neurological tissues).

The drug of choice for treating syphilis is procaine penicillin but, if the patient is allergic to penicillin, erythromycin or a tetracycline may be given instead. As a result of the widespread use of antibiotics to treat the infection, it is rare for patients to progress to the tertiary stage of the disease.

The number of cases of gonorrhoea has continued to rise since the late 1990s. The infection is extremely contagious and the following are the main sites that become contaminated:

- Genitourinary tract
- Rectum
- Tonsils
- Conjunctival sac
- Pharynx.

It is more or less exclusively transmitted through sexual contact. Men who are infected with gonorrhoea are predominantly young heterosexuals, bisexuals and homosexuals. There are many long-term complications associated with this infection and, as such, nurses must endeavour to develop and build upon current STI prevention strategies if the number of cases of gonorrhoea (and other STIs) is to fall.

Caring for patients with STIs demands that the nurse be sensitive to the patient's condition. The nurse is in an ideal position to help relieve the patient's feelings of guilt and anxiety. The social stigma attached to STIs requires that the nurse ensures maintenance of confidentiality at all times. A detailed patient history is needed and the nurse must develop his or her history-taking technique to elicit as much information from the patient as possible. An in-depth physical examination is also needed to ascertain the extent of the disease.

Partner notification (contact tracing) is an important aspect of the management of patients with any STI, because often the sexual partner of the patient with an STI may not have any symptoms. In a GUM clinic, the health adviser usually undertakes this role. Often patients find it difficult or embarrassing to tell their partner that they have an STI; in this case the health adviser may be the best person to do this.

References

Acheson D (1998) Independent Enquiry into Inequalities in Health Report. London: The Stationery Office.

Adler MW (2000) ABC of Sexually Transmitted Diseases, 4th edn. London: BMJ Books.

Aggleton P, Homans H (1987) Educating About AIDS. Bristol: NHS Training Authority.

Arrhigi HM, Guess HA, Metter EJ, Fozard JL (1990) Symptoms and signs of prostatism as risk factors for prostatic surgery. Prostate 16: 253–261.

Ashton J, Seymour H (1991) The New Public Health, 3rd edn. Milton Keynes: Open University Press.

Astbury-Ward E (2000) The erectile dysfunction revolution. Nursing Standard 15(1): 34–40.

Audit Commission (1993) What Seems to be the Matter: Communication between hospitals and patients. London: HMSO.

Baker P (2001) The state of men's health. Men's Health Forum. 1(1): 6–7.

Banks I (2002) Old dogs, new tricks. Men's Health Forum 1(3): 67.

Birth Control Trust and Family Planning Association (1984) Men, Sex and Contraception. London: Birth Control Trust.

Blasko JC, Fowler FJ, Grimm PD, Ragde H (1995) Prostate specific antigen based disease control following ultra sound guided 125 iodine implantation for stage T1/T2 prostatic carcinoma. Journal of Urology 154: 1096–1099.

Blumenfeld AJ, Fleshner N, Casselman B, Trachtenberg J (2000) Nutritional aspect of prostate cancer: A review. Canadian Journal of Urology 1: 927–935

Bostwick DG, Brewer MK (1987) Prostatic intraepithelial neoplasia and early invasion in prostate cancer. Cancer 59: 778–794.

Bott SRJ, Kirby RS (2002) Benign prostatic hyperplasia: Diagnosis and management. Men's Health Journal 1(2): 38–42.

Brechin A, Swain J (1987) Changing Relationships – Shared Action Planning with People with a Mental Handicap. London: Harper & Row.

Bremmer A, Radcliffe K (1993) Missing the diagnosis of neurosyphilis. Journal of Sexual Medicine May/June: 14.

Brown B, Lunt F (1992) Evaluating a 'well man clinic'. Health Visitor 65(1): 12–14.

Buggins E (1995) Mind your language. Nursing Standard 10(1): 21–22.

Calman K (1993) On the State of Public Health. London: HMSO.

Camden and Islington Community Health Service NHS Trust (1998) Positive About Drugs. London: Camden and Islington Community Health Service NHS Trust.

Cancer Research Campaign (1991) Testicular Cancer: Factsheet 16. London: CRC.

Cancer Research Campaign (1998a) Fact Sheet 1: Incidence UK. London: CRC.

Cancer Research Campaign (1998b) Fact Sheet 16.6: Testicular Cancer UK. London: CRC.

Cancer Research Campaign (2001) Scientific Year Book 2001–2002. London: Cancer Research Campaign.

Cancer Research UK (2002) Cancer Stats – Prostate Cancer – UK. London: Cancer Research UK.

CancerBACUP (1999) Understanding Radiotherapy. London: CancerBACUP.

CancerBACUP (2001) Understanding Chemotherapy. London: CancerBACUP.

Caplan P (1987) The Cultural Construction of Sexuality. London: Routledge.

Caplan R, Holland R (1990) Rethinking health education theory. Health Education Journal 49: 10–12.

Carey P, Charlton A, Sloper P, While D (1995) Cancer education in secondary schools. Education Review 47(1): 101–111.

Carr LT (1991) Sexuality: A topical issue for nursing. Nursing Standard 6(1): 52–55.

Carr LT (1995) Sexuality and people with learning disabilities. British Journal of Nursing 4: 1135–1141.

Carson CC (1999) Male sexual dysfunction: diagnosis and treatment of erectile dysfunction. In: Kirby RS, Kirby MG, Farah RN (eds), Men's Health. Oxford: Isis Medical Media, pp. 125–136.

Cates W, Wasserheit JN (1991) Genital chlamydial infections: Epidemiology and reproductive sequelae. American Journal of Obstetrics and Gynecology 164: 1771–1781.

Christ GJ (1995) The penis as a vascular organ. Urologic Clinics of North America 22: 727–745.

Clements S (1991) Male screening: Time waster or life saver? Practice Nurse 4(1): 25–27.

Cole RP (1987) Low back pain and testicular cancer. British Medical Journal 295: 840–841.

Coleman MP, Esteve J, Damiecki P, Arslan A, Renard H (1993) Trends in Cancer Incidence and Mortality. IARC Scientific Publication No. 121. Lyon: IARC.

Communicable Disease Surveillance Centre (2000) Increased transmission of syphilis in Brighton and greater Manchester among men who have sex with men. Communicable Disease Report Weekly 10(43): 383–386.

Communicable Disease Surveillance Centre (2001) Sexually transmitted infections. Quarterly report: Genital chlamydial infection in the United Kingdom. Communicable Diseases Report Weekly 11(26).

Connell R (1995) Masculinities. Cambridge: Polity Press.

Cook N (2000) Testicular cancer: Testicular self examination and screening. British Journal of Nursing 9(9): 338–343.

Coulter A, Entwistle V, Gilbert D (1998) Informing Patients: An assessment of the quality of patient information materials. London: King's Fund.

Creager JG (1983) Human Anatomy and Physiology. Belmont, Calif: Wadsworth Publishing Co.

Curtis H, Hoolaghan T, Jewitt C (eds) (1996) Sexual Health Promotion in General Practice. Oxford: Radcliffe.

Davidson N (2001) Guidelines for practice. In: Davidson N, Lloyd, T (eds), Promoting Men's Health: A guide for practitioners. Edinburgh: Baillière Tindall, pp. 261–287.

Davidson N, Lloyd T (eds) (2001) Promoting Men's Health: A guide for practitioners. Edinburgh: Baillière Tindall.

Dean J, Gingel JC, Wright P, Barnes T (1999) Guidance on the management of erectile dysfunction in primary care. Prescriber suppl 3.

Delaney F (1996) Theoretical issues in intersectoral collaboration. In: Scriven A, Orme J (eds), Health Promotion Professional Perspectives. Basingstoke: Macmillan Press.

Denny E, Jacob F (1990) Defining health promotion. Senior Nurse 10(9): 7–9.

Department for Education and Employment (2000) Sex and Relationship Education Guidance. Nottingham: Department for Education and Employment.

Department of Health (1992) The Health of the Nation. London: HMSO.

Department of Health (1997) The New NHS. London: The Stationery Office.

Department of Health (1998) The Independent Inquiry into Inequalities in Health (Chair Sir Donald Acheson). London: The Stationery Office.

Department of Health (1999a) Our Healthier Nation. London: The Stationery Office.

Department of Health (1999b) Saving Lives: Our Healthier Nation. London: The Stationery Office.

Department of Health (2000a) The NHS Plan: A plan for investment, a plan for reform. London: The Stationery Office.

Department of Health (2000b) The NHS Cancer Plan: A plan for investment. A plan for reform. London: The Stationery Office.

Department of Health (2000c) The NHS Prostate Cancer Programme. London: The Stationery Office.

Department of Health (2001) The National Strategy for Sexual Health and HIV. London: The Stationery Office.

Department of Health and HM Prison Service (2001a) Prison Health Policy Unit and Task Force: Prison health handbook. London: The Stationery Office.

Department of Health and HM Prison Service (2001b) Prison Health Policy Unit and Task Force: Annual Report 2000/2001. London: The Stationery Office.

Department of Health and Social Security (1983) NHS Management Enquiry (the Griffiths Report). London: The Stationery Office.

DeVille-Almond J (2002) Innovations in men's health: Working outside the box. Men's Health Forum 1(3): 88–90.

Dieckmann KP, Pichlmeier U (1997) The prevalence of familial testicular cancer: an analysis of two patient populations and a review of the literature. Cancer 80(10): 1954–1960.

Division of Public Health and Primary Care, University of Oxford (1998) The DISCERN Handbook: Quality criteria for consumer health information. Oxford: Radcliffe Medical Press.

Donovan JL, Frankel SJ, Faulkner A, Selly S (1999) Dilemmas in treating early prostate cancer: The evidence and a questionnaire survey of consultant urologists in the United Kingdom. British Medical Journal 318: 299–300.

Downey P (ed.) (2000a) The prostate. In: An Introduction to Urological Nursing. London: Whurr pp. 82–97.

Downey P (2000b) The penis and urethra. In: Downey P (ed.), Introduction to Urological Nursing. London: Whurr, pp. 98–110.

Downey P, Dean M, Hayes J (1997) Perfect timing. Nursing Times 93(5): 89–90.

Downie RS, Tannahill C, Tannahill A. (1996) Health Promotion Models and Values, 2nd edn. Oxford: Oxford Medical Publications.

Drever F, Whitehead M (1997) Health Inequalities: Decennial Supplement: DS Series No 15. London: The Stationery Office.

Dunn KM, Croft PR, Hackett GI (1998) Sexual problems: A study of the prevalence and need for health care in the general population. Family Practice 15: 519–524.

Edley N, Wetherell M (1995) Men in Perspective: Practice, power and identity. London: Prentice Hall.

Edwards M, Turp G, Crutchley J (1999) Men's Health. In: Edwards M (ed.), The Informed Practice Nurse. London: Whurr, pp. 139–174.

Edwards T (1997) Men in the Mirror: Men's fashion, masculinity and consumer society. London: Cassell.

Erectile Dysfunction Alliance (1999) UK Management Guidelines for Erectile Dysfunction. London: Royal Society of Medicine Press.

Erectile Dysfunction in Primary Care Programme (1999) Nurse Education in Erectile Dysfunction. Module 1. London: Pfizer Ltd.

Erectile Dysfunction in Primary Care Programme (2000) Nurse Education in Erectile Dysfunction. Module 2. London: Pfizer Ltd.

Eurosurveillance (2001) Volume 6(5): 69–90.

Evans G (1994) A history of sexually transmitted diseases. Nursing Times 90(18): 29–31.

Ewels L, Simnett I (1999) Promoting Health: A practical guide, 4th edn. Edinburgh: Scutari Press.

Fareed A (1994) Equal rights for men. Nursing Times 90(5): 26–29.

Feldman HA, Goldstein T, Hatzicristou DO, Krane RJ, Mcinlay JE (1994) Impotence and its medical and social correlates: Results of a Massachusetts male ageing study. Journal of Urology 151: 54–61.

Ferlay J, Bray F, Pisani P, Parkin DM (2001) Globocan 2000: Cancer Incidence, Mortality and Prevalence Worldwide, Version 1.0. IARC Cancer Base No 5. Lyon: IARC Press.

Fillingham S, Douglas J (1997a) Urological Nursing, 2nd edn. London: Baillière Tindall.

Fillingham S, Douglas J (eds.) (1997b) Urological cancers. In: Urological Nursing, 2nd edn. London: Baillière Tindall, pp. 252–284.

Fletcher R (1997) Report on Men's Health Services. University of Newcastle, New South Wales: New South Wales Department of Health.

Fogel CI (1990) Human sexuality and health care. In: Fogel CI, Lauver D (eds), Sexual Health Promotion, pp. 1–38. Philadelphia: WB Saunders.

Forster D, Pannell D, Edwards E (1999) Health Promotion. In Edwards M (ed.), The Informed Practice Nurse. London: Whurr Publications, pp 100–138.

Fulcher J, Scott J (1999) Sociology. Oxford: Oxford University Press.

Furber C (1999) Promoting health to men. In: Harrison T, Dignan K (eds), Men's Health: An introduction for nurses and health professionals. Edinburgh: Churchill Livingstone, pp. 191–219.

Garrett L (1994) The Coming Plague. London: Penguin.

Gelbart M (1999) Casting a long shadow – the sexually transmitted disease in history. In: Weston A (ed.), Sexually Transmitted Infections: A guide to care. London: Nursing Times Books, pp. 1–7.

Goldstein I (1996) Arterial revascularization procedures. Seminal Urology 4: 252–258.

Greenlee RT, Hill-Hammond MB, Murray T, Thun M (2001) Cancer statistics 2001. CA A Cancer Journal for Clinicians 51: 15–36.

Grey A (1993) Speaking of Sex. London: Cassell.

Guly HR (1996) History Taking, Examination, and Record Keeping in Emergency Medicine. Oxford: Oxford University Press.

Harrison T, Dignan K (1999) Men's Health: An introduction for nurses and health professionals. Edinburgh: Churchill Livingstone.

Hartmann U (1998) The efficacy of psychosexual therapy for erectile dysfunction: a critical review of outcome studies. International Journal of Impotence Research 10(suppl 3).

Hawkes T (1972) Metaphor. London: Methuen.

Health Development Agency (2001) Boys' and Young Men's Health. London: Health Development Agency.

Health Education Authority (1992) Chlamydia and NSU: What they are and what you can do about them. London: Health Education Authority

Health Education Authority (1997) Health Related Resources for Older People. London: Health Education Authority.

Healton CG, Messeri P (1993) The effect of video interventions on improving knowledge and treatment compliance in sexually transmitted diseases clinic. Sexually Transmitted Disease 20(2): 70–76.

Hearn J (1994) Research in men and masculinities: Some sociological issues and possibilities. Australian and New Zealand Journal of Sociology 30: 47–70.

Heath H, McCormack B (2002) Nurses, the body and bodywork. In: Heath H, White I (eds), The Challenge of Sexuality in Health Care. Oxford: Blackwell, pp 66–86.

Helman CG (1996) Culture, Health and Illness, 3rd edn. Oxford: Butterworth-Heinemann.

Hendry WF (1999) Testicular cancer. In: Kirby RS, Kirby MG, Farah RN (eds), Men's Health. Oxford: Isis Medical Media, pp. 25–31.

Herrmann B, Johnsson A, Mardh PA (1991) A retrospective study of efforts to diagnose infections by Chlamydia trachomatis in a Swedish county. Sexually Transmitted Diseases 18: 233–237.

Horwich A (1991) Testicular Cancer: Investigation and management. London: Chapman & Hall.

Horwich A, Brada M, Nicholls JEA (1989) Intensive induction chemotherapy for poor risk non- seminomatous germ cell tumours. European Journal of Cancer Clinical Oncology 25: 177–184.

Horwich A, Waxman J, Schroder FH (1995) Tumours of the Prostate. Oxford Textbook of Oncology. Oxford: Oxford University Press.

Jadad AR, Gagliardi A (1998) Rating health information on the Internet: Navigating to knowledge or to Babel? Journal of the American Medical Association 279: 611–614.

Jewitt C (1995) The HIV Project: Sexual History Taking in General Practice. London: The HIV Project.

Johnson M (2002) Health checks for hard hats. Men's Health Forum. 1(3): 70.

Jolliff D, Horne AM (1999) Growing up male. In: Horne AM, Kiselica MS (eds), Handbook of Counselling Boys and Adolescent males: A practitioner's guide. Thousand Oaks, Calif: Sage, pp. 3–23.

Jones LJ (1994) The Social Context of Health and Health Work. Basingstoke: Macmillan.

Jones M (1994) Genitourinary medicine. Nursing Times 90(18): 31–33.

Jorgensen N (1990) Clinical and biological significance of carcinoma in situ of the testis. Cancer Surveys 9: 287–302.

Jovanovich JF (1999) Sexually transmitted diseases in men. In: Kirby RS, Kirby MG, Farah RN (eds), Men's Health. Oxford: Isis, pp. 161–184.

Katz RC, Meters K, Wells J (1995) Cancer awareness and self-examination practices in young men and women. Journal of Behavioural Medicine 18: 377–384.

Keene LC, Davies PH (1999) Drug-related erectile dysfunction. Adverse Drug Reaction Toxicological Review 18(1): 5–24.

Kilmartin CT (1994) The Masculine Self. New York: Macmillan.

Kimmel M (1995) Introduction. In: Sabo D, Gordon DF (eds), Men's Health and Illness: Gender, power and the body. London: Sage.

Kinghorn G (2001) A sexual health and HIV strategy for England. British Medical Journal 323: 243–244.

Kirby RS (1999) Male sexual function. In: Tomlinson J (ed.), ABC of Sexual Health. London. BMJ Books, pp 29–34.

Kirby RS, Kirby MG (1999) Impact of prostatic disease on men's health. In: Kirby RS, Kirby MG, Farah RN (eds), Men's Health. Oxford: Isis Press, pp 11–23..

Koshti-Richman A (1996) The role of the nurse in promoting testicular self-examination. Nursing Times 92(33): 40–41.

Kumar P, Clark M (1996) Clinical Medicine, 3rd edn. London: Saunders.

Laker C (1994) Urological Nursing, 4th edn. London: Scutari Press.

Lawler J (1991) Behind the Screens. Melbourne: Churchill Livingstone.

Leiter E, Brendler H (1967) Loss of ejaculation following bi-lateral retroperitoneal lymph node dissection. Journal of Urology 98: 375–378.

Lewis RW, Witherington R (1997) External vacuum therapy for erectile dysfunction: Use and results. World Journal of Urology 15: 78–82.

Lewis T (1998) Unemployment and men's health. Nursing 3(26): 969–971.

Lloyd T (1996) A Review of Men's Health. London: Royal College of Nursing.

Lloyd T, Forrest S (2001) Boy's and Young Men's Health: Literature and practice review. London: NHS Development Agency.

Lobb-Rossini K (1999) Erectile dysfunction and its management. Journal of Community Nursing 13(10): 16–22.

Lockyer R, Gingell JC (1998) Medicated urethral system for erection (MUSE) in the treatment of the soft glans syndrome in patients with penile prostheses. Sexual Dysfunction 1: 129–132.

Long BC, Glazer G (1995) The patient with reproductive problems. In: Long BC, Phipps WJ, Cassmeyer VL (eds), Adult Nursing: A nursing process approach. London: Mosby, pp. 763–809.

Lorig K, Fries J (1995) The Arthritis Help Book, 4th edn. London: Addison Wesley.

Luker K, Caress A (1989) Rethinking patient education. Journal of Advanced Nursing 14: 711–718.

McCance KL, Huether SE (1998) Pathophysiology: The biologic basis for disease in adults and children, 3rd edn. St Louis: Mosby.

Maccoby EE (1998) The Two Sexes: Growing up apart, coming together. Cambridge, Mass: Stanford University Press

Maccoby EE, Jacklin CN (1974) The Psychology of Sex Differences. Stanford, Calif: Stanford University Press.

McKeown T (1976) The Role of Medicine: Dream mirage or nemesis? London: Nuffield Provincial Hospitals Trust.

McMillan A, Scott GR (2000) Sexually Transmitted Infections. Edinburgh: Churchill Livingstone.

Martin E (1989) The Woman in the Body: A cultural analysis of reproduction. Buckingham: Open University Press.

Mason MD (1996) Tumour markers. In: Horwich A (ed.), Testicular Cancer Investigation and Management, 2nd edn. London: Chapman & Hall, pp. 35–51.

Maynard M (1999) Gender relations. In: Taylor S (ed.), Sociology: Issues and debates. London: Palgrave, pp. 116–135.

Mebust WK, Holtgrewe HL, Cockett ATK (1989) Transurethral prostatectomy: Immediate and post operative complications. A co-operative study of 13 participating institutions evaluating 3885 patients. Journal of Urology 41: 243–247.

Men's Health Forum (2001) National Strategy for Sexual Health and HIV: The Response of the Men's Health Forum. London: Men's Health Forum.

Meryn MD (2002) The time is right: Developing men's health internationally. Men's Health Journal 1(3): 76.

Morello JA, Mizer HE, Wilson ME, Granato PA (1998) Microbiology in Patient Care, 6th edn. Boston: McGraw-Hill.

Moynihan C (1987) Testicular cancer: The psychosocial problems of patients and their relatives. Cancer Survey 6: 477–510.

Moynihan C (1998) Theories in health care and research: Theories of masculinity. British Medical Journal 317: 1072–1075.

Mulhall A (2001) Epidemiology. In: Naidoo J, Wills J (eds), Health Studies: An introduction. London: Palgrave, pp. 39–68.

Naidoo J, Wills J (1994) Health Promotion: Foundations for practice. London: Baillière Tindall.

Naidoo, J, Wills J (2000) Health Promotion: Foundations for practice, 2nd edn. Edinburgh: Baillière Tindall.

National Institutes of Health (1993) NIH consensus development panel on impotence. Consensus Conference on Impotence. Journal of American Medical Association 270: 83–90.

Neal AJ, Hoskin PJ (1997) Clinical Oncology: Basic principles and practice, 2nd edn. London: Arnold.

Nursing and Midwifery Council (NMC) (2002) Code of Professional Conduct. London: NMC.

O'Dowd T, Jewell T (1998) Men's Health. Oxford: Oxford University Press.

O'Leary S (2001) Getting Men to See the Doctor. Men's Health Tackling the Inequalities: Report of a one-day multi-disciplinary conference. London: Men's Health Forum.

Office for National Statistics (2000/2001) Source Labour Force Survey. London: The Stationery Office.

Office for National Statistics (2001) Social Focus on Men. London: The Stationery Office.

Office for National Statistics: General Practice Research Data (1998) Key Health Statistics from General Practice. London: The Stationery Office.

Orchid Cancer Appeal (1997) Testicular Cancer: Awareness leaflet. London: Orchid Cancer Appeal.

Organization of Economic Co-operation and Development (2000) Literacy Skills for the Knowledge Society: Further Results from the International Adult Literacy Survey. London. OECD.

Paolozzi H (1994) Looking after your kit. Nursing Times 90(5): 30–31.

Parkin DM (2001) Global cancer statistics in the year 2000. Lancet Oncology 2: 533–543.

Peate I (1997) Testicular cancer: The importance of effective health education. British Journal of Nursing 6: 311–316

Peate I (1998) Syphilis: Signs, symptoms, treatment and nursing management. British Journal of Nursing 7: 817–823.

Peplau H (1952) Interpersonal Relations in Nursing. New York: Springer.

Perring M, Moran J (1995) Holistic approach to the management of erectile disorders in male sexual health clinic. British Journal of Clinical Practice 49(3): 140–144.

Pimenta J, Fenton KA (2001) Recent trends in Chlamydia trachomatis in the United Kingdom and the potential for national screening. Euro Surveillance 6(6): 81–84.

Pleck J (1981) The Myth of Masculinity. Boston, Mass: MIT Press.

Positive Treatment News (2000) Dr Fax no. 79. Positive Treatment News issue 8 May/June p 15.

Public Health Laboratory Service (2001) Sexually Transmitted Infections in the UK: New episodes seen at genitourinary medicine clinics, 1995–2000. London: PHLS.

Public Health Laboratory Service (2002) Data on STI's in the United Kingdom (1995–2000). London: PHLS.

Quinn M, Babb P, Brock A, Kirby L, Jones J (2001) Cancer Trends in England and Wales, 1950–1999. Studies on Medical and Population Subjects, No 66. London: The Stationery Office.

Raven RW (1994) An Atlas of Oncology. London: Parthenon.

Read G, Stenning SP, Cullen MH (1992) Medical research council prospective study of surveillance for stage I testicular teratoma. Journal of Clinical Oncology 10: 1762–1768.

Reeve S (2002) Sex education takes to the road. Nursing Times 98(5): 36–37.

Riley A (2001) Erectile disorder is a symptom, not a diagnosis. Men's Health Journal 1(1): 8–12.

Robertson S (1995) Men's health promotion in the UK: A hidden problem. British Journal of Nursing 4(7): 382–401.

Robinson KM, Huether SE (1998) Structure and function of the reproductive systems. In: McCance KL, Huether SE (eds) Pathophysiology: The biologic basis for disease in adults and children, 4th edn. St Louis: Mosby, pp. 707–742.

Rooney G, Robinson A (1997) Lookout for the hidden STD. Practitioner 241: 260–263.

Roper N, Logan WW, Tierney A (1996) The Elements of Nursing: A model for nursing based on a model of living, 4th edn. Edinburgh: Churchill Livingstone.

Rosella JD (1994) Testicular cancer health education: An integrative review. Journal of Advanced Nursing 20: 666–671.

Royal College of Nursing (2000) Sexuality and Sexual Health in Nursing Practice. London: Royal College of Nursing.

Sabo D, Gordon DF (1995) Men's Health and Illness: Gender, power and the body. London: Sage.

Salmond A (1982) Theoretical landscapes: On cross-cultural conceptions of knowledge. In: Parkin D (ed.), Semantic Anthropology. London: Academic Press.

Savage J (1995) Nursing Intimacy: An ethnographic approach to nurse–patient interaction. London: Scutari.

Scherer JC, Timby BK (1995) Introduction to Medical–Surgical Nursing. Philadelphia: Lippincott.

Scottish Cancer Intelligence Unit (2000) Trends in Cancer Survival in Scotland 1971–1995. Edinburgh: Information and Statistics Division.

Seedhouse D (1986) Health: The foundations of achievement. Chichester: John Wiley & Sons.

Sharpe RM, Skakkebaek NE (1993) Are oestrogens involved in falling sperm counts and disorders of the male reproductive tract? The Lancet 341: 1392–1395.

Sheerin F, Sine D (1999) Marginalisation and its effects on the sexually-related potentials of the learning-disabled person. Journal of Learning Disabilities for Nursing, Health and Social Care 3(1): 39–49.

Smeltzer SC, Bare BG (2000) Textbook of Medical Surgical Nursing, 9th edn. Philadelphia, Pa: Lippincott.

Smith C, Lloyd B (1978) Maternal behaviour and perceived sex of infant: Revisited. Child Development 49: 1263–1265.

Spark RF (2000) Sexual Health for Men: The complete guide. Mass: Perseus Publishing.

Stamm WE, Guinan ME, Johnson C (1984) Effects of treatment regimens for *Neisseria gonorrhoeae* on simultaneous infection with *Chlamydia trachomatis*. New England Journal of Medicine 310: 545–549.

Stanway A (1995) Sexuality and Cancer: A guide for people with cancer and their partners. London: CancerBACUP.

Steege JF, Stout A, Carson CC (1986) Patient/partner satisfaction. Archives of Sexual Behaviour 15: 393–399.

Stokes T (1997) Screening for chlamydia in general practice: Literature review and summary of the evidence. Journal of Public Health Medicine 19: 227–232.

Stoltenberg J (1989) Refusing to be a Man: Essays on sex and justice. Portland: Breitenbush.

Sutherland C (2001) Women's Health: A handbook for nurses. Edinburgh: Churchill Livingstone.

Sutherland E (1996) Day Surgery: A handbook for Nurses. London: Baillière Tindall.

Swerdlow AJ, dos Santos Silva IM (1983) The Atlas of Cancer Incidence of England and Wales 1968–1978. London: John Wiley

Taylor-Robinson D (1996) Tests for infection with Chlamydia trachomatis. International Journal of STDs and AIDS 7: 19–26.

Tibblin G, Wellin L, Bergstrom R, Ronquist G, Norlen BJ, Adami HO (1995) The value of prostate specific antigen in early diagnosis of prostate cancer: The study of men born in 1913. Journal of Urology 154: 1386–1389.

Tones K, Tilford S (1994) Health Education: Effectiveness, efficiency, and equity, 2nd edn. London: Chapman & Hall.

Tortora GJ, Grabowski SR (1996) Principles of Anatomy and Physiology, 8th edn. New York: Harper Collins

Townsend P, Davidson N, Whitehead M (1988) Inequalities in Health: The Black Report and the health divide. London: Penguin.

Turner D (1995) Testicular cancer and the value of self-examination. Nursing Times 91(1): 30–31.

UK Testicular Cancer Study Group (1994) Aetiology of testicular cancer: Association with congenital abnormalities, age at puberty, infertility and exercise. British Medical Journal 308: 1393–1399

UKCC (1998) Guidelines for Records and Record Keeping. London: UKCC.

Valenis B (1992) Epidemiology and Health Care. Norwalk, Conn: Appleton Lang.

Van Ooijen E (1995) How illness may affect a patient's sexuality? Nursing Times 91: 36–37.

Wagner G, Saenz de Tejada I (1998) Update on male erectile dysfunction. British Journal of Medicine 316: 678–682.

Walsh M (1997) Watson's Clinical Nursing and Related Sciences, 5th edn. London: Baillière Tindall

Wardle J, Steptoe A, Burckhardt R, Vogele C, Vila J, Zarczynski Z (1995) Testicular self-examination: Attitudes and practices among young men in Europe. Preventive Medicine 23: 206–210.

Watson C (2001) Well man clinics. In: Davidson N, Lloyd T (eds), Promoting Men's Health: A guide for practitioners. Edinburgh: Baillière Tindall, pp. 165–175.

Watson J (2000) Male Bodies: Health, culture and identity. Buckingham: Open University Press.

Webb CA (1999) Men's health: The background. In: Harrison T, Dignan K (eds), Men's Health: An introduction for nurses and health professionals. Edinburgh: Churchill Livingstone, pp. 1–14.

Weeks J (1993) Sexuality. London: Routledge.

Weston A (1999) Striking back at syphilis. In: Weston, A. (ed.), Sexually Transmitted Infections: A guide to care. London: Nursing Times Books, pp. 13–21.

Wheeler PN (2001) Sexuality: Meaning and relevance to learning disabilities nurses. British Journal of Nursing 10: 920–927.

Whitehead M (1988) The health divide. In: Townsend P, Davidson N, Whitehead M (eds), Inequalities in Health: The Black Report and the health divide, 2nd edn. London: Penguin.

WHO (1986) Ottawa Charter for Health Promotion: An International Conference on Health Promotion. Geneva: WHO.

Williamson P (1995) Their own worst enemy. Nursing Times 91(48): 25–27.

Wilton T (2000) Sexualities in Health and Social Care. Buckingham: Open University Press.

Wisdom A (1992) A Colour Atlas of STDs. London: Wolfe's Medical Publications.

World Health Organization (1975) Education and Trends in Human Sexuality – the training of health professionals. WHO. Teaching Report Series No 572. Geneva: WHO.

Glossary

Accountability: the process by which responsibility is publicly addressed and reported on.

Active listening: observing and interpreting a person's non-verbal behaviour, as well as listening and interpreting the person's verbal messages.

Aetiology: assigning a cause to a particular outcome. The aetiology of sexually transmitted infections, for example, may be attributed to the non-use of condoms.

Androgen: hormone secreted by the testes and adrenal cortex.

Benign: a pattern of tumour growth characterized by uncontrolled cellular division, remaining localized. There is no invasion of surrounding tissues or metastases.

Cancer: a generic term used to describe any malignant tumour.

Carcinoma: a malignant tumour of epithelial tissue.

Class: the division and ranking of groups of people depending on occupational role, which arose during the growth and development of capitalism. Social class is concerned with status and power as well as income. The Registrar General in the Government surveys measures of class based on occupation.

Cremaster muscles: a small band of skeletal muscle found in the spermatic cord; elevates the testes on sexual arousal or during exposure to cold.

Cryptorchidism: a condition whereby the testes do not descend into the scrotal sac.

Culture: a way of life including values and beliefs, and customs, as well as social and family arrangements.

Dartos muscle: muscle found in the subcutaneous tissue of the scrotum; during contraction causes wrinkling of the scrotal skin.

Detumescence: subsidence from swelling.

Differentiation: a process that involves dividing cells maintaining a degree of morphological and biochemical similarity to their parental cell type. Loss of

156

differentiation is a distinguishing feature of cancer cells, which may be highly differentiated and therefore very different from their cells or the tissue of origin. Generally, the higher the level of differentiation, the poorer the prognosis.

Dorsal: pertaining to the back or posterior; opposite of ventral.

Ejaculation: the release of seminal fluid.

Emission: a discharge, particularly of semen.

Ethnicity: features of social life, e.g. culture, religion, history and language, which are shared by groups of people and passed down to the next generation.

Empowerment: to encourage and enable others to feel in control of their own state of affairs and to have a say in their own lives and destinies.

Epidemiology: the study of how diseases are distributed among diverse groups of people and the factors that affect this distribution.

Erection: the enlargement and stiffening of the penis, resulting from the engorgement of the spongy erectile tissue with blood.

Gender: the social meaning and value of the difference between the sexes. Gender is associated with socially ascribed attributes, features and roles that are seen as belonging to either males or females. Social role that is bound up with being biologically male or female.

Hydronephrosis: dilatation of the pelvis and calyces of either one or both kidneys, resulting from obstruction to the flow of urine.

Incidence: the number of new cases that occur in a specific group of individuals (population) over an interval of time.

Leydig cells: these cells produce the chief androgen – testosterone.

Libido: conscious or unconscious sexual desire.

Lifestyle: manner of living often thought of as being chosen by the individual, e.g. whether to smoke or to exercise. Also affected by social factors, e.g. income.

Lymphoma: a malignant condition of the lymph tissue.

Malignant: a pattern of tumour growth characterized by uncontrolled cellular division; invasion of the surrounding tissues usually associated with metastatic spread.

Mechanoreceptors: a sensory receptor that responds to pressure, touch or other mechanical stimulation.

Morbidity: relating to a disease or abnormal or disordered condition. Morbidity measures the amount of illness or disease in a population.

Mortality rates: these are the numbers of deaths within the population. To measure crude mortality, take the total number of deaths in the population and divide by the population size.

Nocturia: excessive urination at night.

Orchidectomy: removal of one or both testes.

Organic: relating to an organ.

Orgasm: the culmination of sexual intercourse.

Pathogenic: disease producing, e.g. a term applied to bacteria.

Plaque: a patch or small differentiated area on a body surface, e.g. skin or mucosa.

Prevalence: the size of a defined population that is experiencing a condition over a given period or at a specific point in time.

Proximal: nearer the attachment of a limb to the trunk, or nearer to the point of origin or attachment.

Prosthesis: fabricated substitute for a diseased or missing part of the body, e.g. the testicle.

Psychogenic: of mental origin or causation.

Risk factors: those factors that make an individual or a group of individuals (the population) susceptible to a disease or illness. These factors may be genetic, e.g. a familial history of breast cancer.

Screening: the assumptive identification of a disease or condition through the use of tests, e.g. analysis of prostate-specific antigen to identity those men who may be at risk of developing prostate cancer.

Seminoma: a malignant tumour of the testes.

Social inequalities: these inequalities are associated with access to resources, power, status and income. Social processes and institutions have the power to produce, reproduce and maintain these components.

Socialization: the process by which the individual is adapted to his social environment and becomes a recognized, co-operating and efficient member of it.

Stigma: a mark of shame or discredit.

Spermatozoa: mature male reproductive cells.

Staging: an internationally agreed measuring system for cancer that considers the tumour's size, the presence or location of affected lymph nodes, and the absence or presence of metastases.

Strata: layers of differential tissue, the aggregate of which forms any given structure, e.g. the prostate gland.

Teratoma: usually a benign tumour containing the three primary germ layers.

Tumescence: swelling, inflation.

Tumour: a distinct region of growth deregulation, resulting in a dividing colony of cells of varying size; this may display either malignant or benign characteristics.

Ventral: pertaining to the anterior or front side of the body; the opposite of dorsal.

Index